Dr. Jordan Metzl's
RUNNING STRONG

Also by Dr. Jordan Metzl

The Young Athlete

The Athlete's Book of Home Remedies

The Exercise Cure

Dr. Jordan Metzl's
RUNNING STRONG

THE SPORTS DOCTOR'S COMPLETE GUIDE TO STAYING HEALTHY AND INJURY-FREE FOR LIFE

Jordan D. Metzl, MD
with Claire Kowalchik

Rodale books may be purchased for business or promotional use or for special sales. For information, please write to: Special Markets Department, Rodale, Inc., 733 Third Avenue, New York, NY 10017

Runner's World is a registered trademark of Rodale Inc.

Printed in the United States of America

Rodale Inc. makes every effort to use acid-free ∞, recycled paper ♻.

Exercise illustrations by Kagan McLeod; anatomy illustrations by Primal Pictures
Book design by Christina Gaugler

Library of Congress Cataloging-in-Publication Data is on file with the publisher

ISBN 978–1–62336–459–5   trade paperback

Distributed to the trade by Macmillan

2   4   6   8   10   9   7   5   3   1   trade paperback

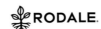

We inspire and enable people to improve their lives and the world around them.
rodalebooks.com

Every morning around the world alarms ring at 5:30 a.m. In every country, in every bed, athletes debate with themselves: Do I hit the snooze button, or do I swing my feet over the side of the bed and go running?

This book is dedicated to the millions of runners who, against all logic, suppress the desire to stay in bed. They kick off the covers and swing their legs around to hit the floor.

May the knowledge in these pages and videos keep you moving ahead with health and enthusiasm for many years to come.

CONTENTS

PART III: GETTING THE MOST FROM YOUR MACHINE

PART IV: TOOLS OF THE TRADE

PART V: HIS AND HERS

STEP INTO MY OFFICE

Why do you run?

Because it feels good.

Because it lowers your risk of heart disease, diabetes, cancer.

Because it relieves stress and eases depression.

Because running builds your fitness for hiking tough trails or playing capture the flag with your kids.

Because as a runner you can eat pie.

Because you love busting all out for a PR in a 5-K.

Because you love meeting the edge in a marathon, an ultra, or a tri and pushing past it.

Because you love joining the moving party on the road at your hometown 5-miler.

Because it fills you with energy.

Because it makes you happier.

Because it makes you brave.

Because it makes you feel good about yourself.

I hear so many answers to this simple question. And what I hear that's common to all of those answers is that running is important to you, it's important to your best life.

I get that, because running is important to my best life too. And it has been for many years. I exercise every day. Why? I have more energy, more focus in everything I do, more motivation. And I love to compete. As a 32-time (and still counting) marathoner and 12-time Ironman triathlete who has saved the date for next year's Ironman Lake Placid, I love to push my limits. But the number one reason I run is the pure joy of movement.

But it's pure hell—physically and emotionally—when you're injured and can't run. I get that too. It's the reason

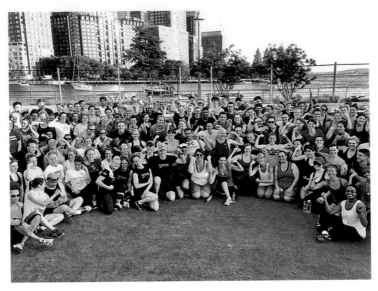

Dr. Metzl and crew at an IronStrength workout in New York City.

I became a sports doc. I know how traumatic it is to be sidelined from the sport you love.

I've been in love with sports ever since I could play football with my brothers in our backyard. In high school it was baseball and soccer, and then in college just soccer. I was physically active every day, and it made me a better student and a happier human being.

Then during my first year of med school at the University of Missouri, at soccer practice, one move changed everything. I'll never forget that day. The sun was shining, the temperature was perfect—cool, but not cold. I was playing striker up front, and as the goalie cleared the ball, I twisted to get it. My knee popped and I went down with excruciating pain. I knew immediately that I had torn my ACL (anterior cruciate ligament), and I was devastated because my sports career, as I knew it then, was over.

I'd defined myself as an athlete virtually my entire life. Sure, I was studying to be a doctor, but a huge piece of me had just been taken away. I didn't know how I would wake up the next day and the next and the next and *not* play sports.

I had surgery and rehabbed my knee, and I worked my way back to sports—to running and triathlons. Along the way I discovered functional strength training, which helped me ease my knee pain. I eventually developed enough strength, after years of doing it, to make me a better athlete than I was before my injury. I took what I learned about strength training and created the IronStrength workout, which I now teach for free to runners and other athletes twice a month to help them get stronger and prevent injury. About 25 people came to my first class. Today I have a listserv with about 6,000 subscribers. In addition to my classes, more than nine million runners around the world have done IronStrength online. It has been tremendously gratifying to see it grow.

I will always remember that loss on the soccer field. And what I can say now is that it was, in a strange way, a gift, and one that keeps on giving. It's what drives me in my medical practice to help my patients. I understand how important movement is to them both physically *and* emotionally, not just

YOUR RUNNER PROFILE	WHAT YOU'LL LEARN (well some of it, because there's a ton of info in this book)
I just got started and I run about 30 minutes three times a week. I run for my health and to keep my weight in check. At this point, I'm testing the waters, so to speak. I don't yet have any long-term plans or goals.	• How to choose the right running shoes and other gear • How to safely increase your mileage • How to know he difference between good and bad pain (yes, there is such a thing as good pain) • How to prevent injury with my IronStrength workout for runners and flexibility training • How to adjust your stride to prevent injury • How to fix an injury if you get one • How to eat to fuel your running and keep your weight where you want it • How to prepare for and run your first race if you want to test those waters too some day
I have been running for several years and put in about 5 miles almost every day. I run because it keeps me sane, and I know that it's good for my health. Every now and then I'll enter a race—a 5-K or 10-K—but I'm not a serious competitor.	• How to make sure running is always fun • How my IronStrength workout can keep you injury-free • How to fix an injury if you get one • Why you should use a foam roller every day before and after you run, and how to use it • How to eat to fuel your running, racing, and health
I'm a college student and I run track and cross-country. My right hamstring is my Achilles' heel and I just pulled it.	• How to treat that hamstring injury and make sure it never happens again • How my IronStrength workout can prevent injuries and improve your race times • How to use a foam roller to relax tight muscles and keep you running healthy • How to harness the power of your mind for training and race-day success
I've been running for 5 years. I run about 30 miles a week. I've raced from a 5-K up to a half-marathon, and I really want to tackle the big one—a marathon.	• How to build mileage safely and prepare for your first marathon • How my IronStrength workout can help prevent injury and improve your performance • How to use a foam roller to keep your muscles supple • How to eat to fuel long runs and your marathon • How to run 26.2 miles without bonking • How to harness the power of your mind to master your marathon
I run 35 to 40 miles a week and race everything from a 5-K to a half-marathon. I just learned I'm pregnant and want to keep running during my pregnancy.	• How much mileage is safe for you and your baby • What level of intensity is safe • When to call it quits with running and walk or swim instead • How your nutritional needs change when you are running during pregnancy • How pregnancy makes you more vulnerable to injury, and what to do about it • Racing during pregnancy • How to come back to running after pregnancy

YOUR RUNNER PROFILE	WHAT YOU'LL LEARN (well some of it, because there's a ton of info in this book)
I ran cross-country and track in high school and college. I love to race any distance and consider myself a serious competitor. Unfortunately, I seem to be plagued by Achilles problems.	• How to take care of that Achilles so it doesn't keep you off the road, out of training, and on the sideline on race day • How my IronStrength workout can help prevent injury and make you faster • How to use a foam roller to release tightness from your muscles • How to make the most of your physiology for best performance • How to harness the power of your mind for race-day success
I started running in my twenties and loved it. I would run 6 days a week and race everything from 5-Ks to marathons. At 32 I became a mom and that put a serious dent in my mileage. Now my kids are 12 and 14, and I'm working on increasing my weekly mileage and maybe getting back to racing, but right now I have plantar fasciitis and it's killing me.	• How to get rid of that plantar fasciitis once and forever • How the mechanics of a woman's body affect running and can contribute to injury • How to increase mileage and intensity safely • How my IronStrength workout can prevent injury and make you a better runner • Why and how to use a foam roller every day on your muscles • How to choose the best race-training plan for your lifestyle and level of fitness
I'm 67. I've been a runner for 40 years and amassed a bundle of age-group awards at distances from 5-K to the marathon. I've had my share of injuries from running and other sports. Currently everything's working fine, though I have some arthritis in my knees. I simply want to keep running because I love it. It's one of the best parts of my day.	• How to slow the progression of arthritis • How my IronStrength workout can help you manage arthritis and prevent injury • How to use a foam roller to keep your muscles flexible • How to treat an injury if you get one
I love distance and the marathon is my passion. My dream is to qualify for Boston.	• How my IronStrength workout can improve your performance and prevent injury • How to get the most out of your physiology for optimal performance • How to use a foam roller to relieve muscle tightness during heavy training • How to eat and drink to fuel and hydrate your body for long distances • How to avoid bonking in your qualifying marathon • How to harness the power of your mind to help produce your best race

because of that loss on the soccer field but because of what I live today—movement is important physically and emotionally to me too.

Over the years I have developed three separate roles, each of which defines me: sports doctor, athlete, and fitness instructor. I'm all three.

As a sports doctor, I love not only getting my patients and friends back on the road but also helping them get strong, stay strong, and enjoy running for a lifetime. Getting to this point in my career was a marathon of sorts for me. Between college, medical school, residency, and fellowships in sports medicine, I thought I'd never get here. Much like running, I just tried to keep my feet moving, and after many years of training, I'm now in a position to help treat and educate others.

As my medical practice has grown, I feel so blessed to be awarded the opportunity to help people develop active and healthy lifestyles. Being a doctor is about keeping people healthy, and in my opinion the medicine of exercise, and particularly the medicine of running, is the best way to go. I feel so lucky every day at work that I am in a position to help others. Even when my days are long and tough at the office, I get a true sense of gratitude from helping others achieve their goals. The runners who come see me range from high-level runners to beginners looking to complete their first 5-Ks. I see 80-year-olds, teens, and everyone in between, and I view each person as someone I can help make healthier and a better runner. I make fast runners faster and keep veteran runners running, and I get a deep satisfaction no matter whom it is I have helped. I love what I do. And my ultimate goal for my practice, for my Iron-Strength classes, and for this book is to take everyone and get them to a place where over time, no matter who they are, they have learned to take care of themselves.

Now, let's get back to you. What kind of runner are you? And how is this book going to help you?

Part of what I love about my profession is that I get to interact with all kinds of people. I love to talk with runners in my office, listen to their stories, find out what's going on, and then give them not only medical advice but also encouragement to be their healthiest selves and to set goals and go after them. If you live in Burbank, Banff, or Brussels, you're probably not going to come to the Hospital for Special Surgery in New York City, so I am inviting you to step into my office with this book. I created a series of videos with *Runner's World* magazine called "Inside the Doctor's Office" that

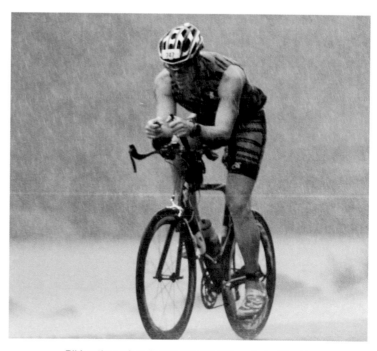

Biking through a downpour at Ironman Lake Placid.

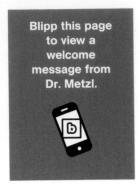

Blipp this page to view a welcome message from Dr. Metzl.

address running injuries as well as your most common questions about running shoes, running form, whether or not to take anti-inflammatories before a race, and more. I filmed this series inside my office in New York City, but the cool thing is that people from anywhere around the world can step into my office 24 hours a day, 7 days a week for a consult with these videos. It's a virtual visit to my office. I show you exactly where injuries occur on Rex the skeleton and on real, live model Meghan, who also demonstrates the IronStrength workout and other exercises that help heal and prevent injuries. You'll be able to access the videos, alongside the in-depth written information, right here from this book. (Technology is a beautiful thing, isn't it?)

Throughout the book, you'll see a little icon that looks like this:

It's your signal that there's a video available relevant to the content on that page. After downloading the free

Blippar application from your mobile device's App store (or Blippar.com), you can then use your phone to scan the page and view the video, stepping into my virtual office. I want your experience with this book to be as personal as possible, because that's how this information will make the most sense and be most beneficial to you. And, hey, it's also more fun that way. I am so excited about this, and I'm sure you will be too. So go download the free Blippar app and test it out right here. Scan this page to view a special message from me.

Welcome to my office!

Wherever you are in the world, I hope that reading *Dr. Jordan Metzl's Running Strong* and watching the videos will help you stay healthy, improve your performance, and become the best runner you can be. Whether you are near or far, thank you so much for being part of my running community.

I look forward to seeing you on the road, my fellow running friends.

With best wishes,
Jordan

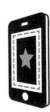

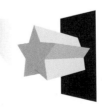

DOWNLOAD ▶ **FILL SCREEN** ▶ **BLIPP PAGE**
BLIPPAR APP   **WITH PAGE**   **INTO LIFE!**

PART I

Nuts and Bolts

Bones, muscles, joints, and tendons: Stack them up, connect them, and you have the human machine. How they're stacked, how they work together, and how you take care of them determine whether you run healthy, strong, and speedy—or not. Let's take a look under the hood.

CHAPTER 1

THE RIGHT STUFF

Ripping my ACL in soccer practice during my med school years was devastating, but I can now say it was the single most important event to influence both my work as a sports physician and how I take care of my own health as a runner and triathlete. Like most people who suffer severe knee injuries, I eventually developed some arthritis. And I'm going to be honest with you: I was worried—was I going to be able to keep running?

When the arthritis showed up, I had been a sports medicine doc for about 10 years. I dug deep into the research and began exploring what I could do as an athlete to manage the pain, stay healthy, and keep running, and I found the answers. Today I can honestly say I am a better, stronger athlete than I was in my twenties before the injury, and I'm a better sports doctor too.

This is where Jordan Metzl the athlete and Dr. Metzl the physician come together. Not only have I researched everything I recommend, but I have also tried it on myself. I want to keep running until I'm 90 and beyond, and I now have the right stuff to do just that. I want to give it to you, so that you too can take the good medicine of running every day and enjoy healthy, injury-free running for the rest of your life.

BELIEVE IT

As I have developed my get-stronger, run-better, stay-injury-free plan, I have shaped a philosophy of exercise that informs everything I do for myself as an athlete as well as the advice I give my patients. That philosophy is built on several principles, rooted in biomechanics and physiology, of how exercise benefits mind and body and what you need to do to keep running in good health. Get to know them, and everything else I'm going to tell you in this book will make sense.

Daily Exercise—Even When You're Injured—Is the Best Medicine

Look, our bodies are made to move. Throughout most of human history, since our hunter-gatherer beginnings, we have exercised every day—stalking prey, running to avoid becoming prey, gathering wild fruits and veggies, and later tilling the soil, tending the herd, milking the cows, pulling in the harvest, grinding grains, kneading bread . . . you get it. Only recently in human history are so many of us sitting on our butts, whether it's in front of the computer doing our jobs or the TV watching our favorite sitcoms, or both. The more you sit, the greater your risk of diabetes and cardiovascular disease and a whole array of other problems. No surprise, right? When you exercise every day, you are preventing serious disease and making your body fitter and stronger for anything and everything you want to do: running, playing with your kids, taking care of your home, traveling around the world. Stay active, stay healthy.

Then there are the benefits to your mind. We all know and love the runner's high, right? But there is so much more. Running energizes your day, makes you more creative, helps you focus, lifts a sagging mood. Regular exercise is literally an antidepressant for many people. Running in the morning also seems to have an additional benefit, turning on your metabolic furnace for the day. The foods you eat during the day are metabolized more quickly and efficiently if you have turned on your metabolic furnace first thing in the morning with a run. I tell my patients, "Give me 30 minutes every morning and I'll give you a healthier life."

Exercise is the best medicine, and I want you to take it every day. I do. Some of you already run every day, or you run every other day or third day and do other stuff in between. Awesome! My goal is to keep you on the road and make you the healthiest runner you can be!

But what about rest and recovery? How do you prevent overtraining if you exercise every day? These are great questions, and here's my answer: Sure, your body needs rest and recovery to respond and rebuild after the trauma of exercise, because while it's good medicine, exercise does temporarily traumatize muscle and bone. It's how you get stronger—breaking down and building up again. But allowing your body to rebuild doesn't mean you need to lie down on the couch with the TV remote in one hand and a bag of chips in the other while repairs are being made. If you run every day, rest and recovery might be a slow 30-minute run the day after an intense speed workout. Or maybe you want to mix it up and cross-train: run hard one day, and then bike or swim or strength-

train the next. I love yoga once a week if you can swing it; data shows it does both mind and body good. The key is to prevent injuries from overuse, also called overtraining injuries. These are by far the most common types of problems that runners encounter and include everything from shin splints to runner's knee to certain types of anemia. Overtraining occurs when you do the same thing at the same high intensity over and over and over again without listening to your body's cues.

Okay, Dr. Metzl, but do you really want me to exercise when I'm injured? Yep. And here's why. First of all, you'll be miserable after a few days of lazing around; your spirit and energy will droop. You'll feel sluggish and tired, grumpy and irritable. Secondly, that speed and endurance you built? It fades away if you sit on your butt—and quickly if you're a beginner.

Now I'm not suggesting that you keep running through the pain—which I know some of you do. I don't want you to do anything that hurts. But I do want you to take the good medicine of exercise every day, especially keeping up with cardio. Bike, swim, run in the pool. The elliptical trainer and ElliptiGO are the most running-specific machines to use when you can't pound the pavement. Find something you like that doesn't aggravate your injury. And stick with strength training: Tendon injuries in particular get better faster with the right strength moves, and strong muscles prevent injury when you get back on the road. The better your conditioning when you return to running, the easier it will be to slip back into training close to where you stopped, and the less likely you will be to reinjure yourself because you lost strength. I call this *dynamic rest*, and throughout this book you'll see my recommendations for how you can keep active every day, even when you are injured.

Think you don't have time to exercise every day? This is the number one reason people give for not exercising regularly—they don't have time. Look, I get it. We all lead incredibly busy lives. We work in an office or at home, we take care of our children, clean, cook, buy groceries, mow the grass, do the laundry; the list goes on and on. And technology has only made us busier because we carry our work around with us on our phones. Plus, we all need to eat, sleep, and steal a little leisure time. Some days when you are just exhausted, the 30-minute sitcom calls to you a lot louder than the 30-minute run. But that 30-minute run

ALL ABOUT RICE

This sports medicine acronym gets thrown at athletes the way the real stuff is tossed at a bride and groom after their wedding—in abundance and because it's the traditional thing to do. Well, as with anything that gets used over and over again, people stop thinking about whether or not it makes good sense. There has also been some enthusiasm for MICE, adding movement to the equation. But tossing mice at the bride and the groom skeeves me out a bit, so I think we'll stick with RICE + active recovery.

RICE stands for rest, ice, compression, and elevation, and here is how you are traditionally supposed to apply it.

- Stop activity
- Ice the injured area a few times a day for the first 2 days after injury to reduce inflammation
- Apply compression, typically by wrapping the area with an elastic compression bandage, to control swelling
- Elevate the injured area above the level of your heart to keep swelling down

Does it work? For certain injuries, yes, with one caveat: that you substitute dynamic rest for complete rest. I want you to move every day. If you can't run with your injury, choose something you *can* do. Swim or bike, and keep up with upper-body strength training. This helps you stay fit, and you will feel good both physically and emotionally.

I love ice. It is Mother Nature's anti-inflammatory and helps reduce pain and swelling. You will see I recommend it throughout this book because it's a great treatment for most injuries.

Compression is great to help reduce postworkout muscle swelling, and some runners believe it quickens recovery. Others swear that it improves performance. My take is that compression is a good thing to try either in the form of compression socks, leggings, or even some of the compression sleeves. If you like compression, so do I!

After your race or tough workout, don't sit around. Active recovery might be a little swim or easy bike ride. Gently moving muscles promotes bloodflow and healing; I'm a fan.

The bottom line: Dynamic RICE can be part of an effective treatment plan for injury.

can give you the mental and physical energy to get more done during the rest of your day so that you can still squeeze in 30 minutes of TV time.

Exercise is so important to your physical health, mental health, happiness, and longevity. Find a spot in your schedule that can be your sacred running space. I go out first thing in the morning and then at the end of my workday. Running in the morning pumps me up for a great day, and after I have seen my patients, exercise clears my head and sets me up for whatever I have scheduled in the evening. For you, maybe your lunch hour is when you can make a consistent commitment. The key is to be honest with yourself about when you'll be most motivated to go out for that 30-minute or hour-long run. If you're not a morning person, trying to get up with the roosters is probably not the best idea. Also, think about the time of day when there's the least likelihood that someone   kid or coworker—might derail you. Finally, don't let anyone interfere. Set boundaries around exercising. If someone pleads with you to have a meeting during your lunch-run hour or your kids beg you to take them to the park, find a compromise that still allows you to run. Hold your run time sacred. This is the best thing you can do for yourself every day—just do it.

The Key to Success Is a Strong Kinetic Chain

You love running, right? Maybe it's the only physical activity you really want to do on a regular basis. And you know that to be good at anything, you need to practice, so to be a better runner, you need to run—absolutely! And that's one excuse runners give for doing no strength training. Then there's this: When your sport of choice involves the great outdoors, sunlight, fresh air, cruisin' down the road, over the trail, or along the beach, who wants to be stuck inside a sweaty, smelly gym doing semi-static strength exercises? I get that. I'm a runner too. But I also want to run for the rest of my life and run to my fullest potential, so I strength-train two or three times a week.

Running is great, but it can create muscle imbalances or accentuate ones you already have. If you have a weak left hip abductor, for example, your left knee may come under extra strain when you run and over time may get injured. Which brings me to one of the most important concepts I want you to take away from this book—the *kinetic chain*. I'm going to talk about this in more detail in the next chapter, but here's the CliffsNotes version: When you run—when you do any kind of movement—multiple muscles, bones, and joints are called on to work together to create fluid motion. Remember that catchy little tune you heard as a kid: "The ankle bone's connected to the shinbone, and the shinbone's connected to the knee bone . . ." and so on? Well, that's how it goes in running: Your feet, lower legs, knees,

Quick Tip: On a Scale of Slim to Stout

As I tell my patients, "I'd much rather you are mild to moderately overweight and active than skinny and inactive." The benefits of activity far outweigh the national obsession with thinness.

thighs, hips, lower back, core, arms, and shoulders are all part of your running kinetic chain, and when one link isn't working, the repercussions can be felt all the way up or down the chain. One weak link forces all the others to work harder, and under too much stress, bad things happen. Weakness isn't just defined by physical strength; flaws in flexibility cause trouble too. For example, too-tight calves will pull excessively on your Achilles tendon, which can cause tendonitis. When you strengthen all the links in the chain and maintain good flexibility from top to bottom, you'll run stronger and stay injury-free.

Isolated, Single-Muscle Exercises Have No Basis in Reality

Now that I have introduced you to the kinetic chain, you will understand why I'm going to tell you to walk right past the exercise machines at the gym. When was the last time you were lying on your back pushing something heavy up over your chest as you do when you bench press? Or better yet, do you ever recall lying on your belly and pulling a weighted object toward your butt with one leg, like you do when you perform hamstring curls? Whether you are running or cleaning up the yard or putting groceries away, you are using your whole body. Many muscles fire simultaneously or in rapid succession along your kinetic chain to create that fluid, beautiful thing we call movement. So

you need to strengthen your muscles in ways that use your whole body and with exercises that *mimic movements you actually do in real life.* This is called functional strength training.

The exercises in my IronStrength workout for runners, which you will find in Chapter 12, do just that. They are full-body exercises and, with the exception of the arm moves, they rely on your body, not weights, for resistance. Plus, there's a bonus: Many of them mimic the movements you use in running, so they build strength right where you need it.

Single-Leg Exercises Build Amazing Strength and Stability

I may not be a fan of single-muscle exercises, but I love single-*leg* moves. Try this right now: Stop reading, get up, and stand on one leg, paying attention to what's going on in your standing leg. Do you feel your muscles working to keep you stable and upright? Now, while still standing on that one leg, move your arms as if you are running and notice how your muscles from your butt to your toes work even harder to keep you balanced. One last little test: Try a one-legged squat. Again, standing on one leg, bend at the knee and lower your body as if you are going to sit down in a chair, keeping your upper body in a more-or-less vertical position and pushing your butt behind you as you lower down. Some of you might be able to do this with ease—congratulations, your strong muscles won't let you down.

Single-leg squats, lunges, and hops build incredible strength and stability. The benefit of great balance isn't just to prevent you from falling on your butt. A stable runner is a healthy runner and a more efficient runner. One of the most important elements of injury-free running is good alignment. When all the links in your kinetic chain are in the right order, your body can better handle the stress of running and more gently absorb ground reaction forces—the forces that drive up your leg when your foot strikes the ground. With strength and stability, you move more efficiently; all your energy is focused forward, in the direction you want to go, instead of being wasted in wiggling hips or wobbly knees.

Finally, think about the stance phase of running: Your foot is planted on the ground, you lower your body, and then you push back up as you go to push off. You are kind of doing a single-leg squat, so including single-leg exercises in your strength workout builds muscles specific to running. Good idea, don't you think?

Strong Butt = Happy Life

The good old gluteus maximus is a runner's best friend. And a lot of us sit on it for way too many hours every day. This is the biggest and strongest muscle in your body. When it hooks up with gluteus medius and gluteus minimus—well, they make a powerful

threesome that generates most of the propulsive force when you run. Your glutes also join forces with your core muscles to provide stability when you run. I love stability in a runner, and you will too, if you don't already.

Here's what happens when you *don't* have stability: As you run, you get too much movement in your hips, too much motion in the ocean; your hips rock up and down. Picture this: As you plant your right foot, let's say, and your right hip drops down, your right knee is forced inward toward your left leg. It's not a pretty picture, and this movement can mess up the tracking of your knee-cap and lead to an injury called runner's knee. It also pulls on your iliotibial band (ITB), a thin band of tissue that runs from your hip joint along the outside of your thigh and attaches just below the knee to your tibia. Over time, pulling a tight ITB over the bony protuberance on the outside of your knee creates soreness in the band called iliotibial band syndrome, which can be a real pain to get rid of. You may even find that the inward movement of your leg causes you to overpronate, which can lead to foot problems, shin issues, and trouble all the way up to your hips. This is your kinetic chain in action—unfortunately, not a positive action. Strengthen that butt and your troubles will disappear.

Strong glutes also produce strong performance. Running economy is a key factor in how fast and far you go; it's all about how you spend the energy

Grace Taylor*: Jumping for Joy

Doing plyometric jump squats makes me all giggly inside. It's the jumping. When as an adult do you get an excuse to jump up and down? Makes me feel like a kid. But most important, it keeps my knees healthy so I can keep running. I have never been hooked on anything before, but now I'm hooked on running.

It all started one spring when the company I work for offered all employees an opportunity to participate in a wellness screening. My results showed that I was overweight, so when it was announced that the company had entered a global corporate fitness challenge—a 16-week competition to see which company could score the most steps—I signed up. I even volunteered to be the team captain, which meant I was responsible for my team's success *and* I needed to be a good role model!

Fortunately, when you work in New York City, you walk everywhere. But I travel to California often for business and the cities there aren't as walkable, so I needed something else. Running! I decided to train for a half-marathon and signed up for one that fall.

As the race approached, I could feel things getting tense in my knees, but I ran anyway and finished. Afterward I couldn't even walk a block. And that's when I went to see Dr. Metzl, who diagnosed runner's knee. He advised that I use a foam roller to work out tightness in my muscles and that I also begin plyometric jump squats once I was able. With the foam roller, I improved very quickly and could run again in a week.

At the same time that I added running to my life, I made a decision to eat more healthfully. I follow two big rules: only have dessert on Saturdays, and eat a pile of green things whenever possible (you can have an enormous pile of green things and consume very few calories).

By having dessert once a week, I avoid feeling deprived, and it gives me an out in social settings where there's pressure to have dessert. My boyfriend and I make dessert a celebration at the end of the week. We get something special and savor every bite.

Since I started running and eating better, I'm much happier. At the time of the wellness screening, I weighed 170 pounds; by the end of the summer, I was 140—less than what I weighed in college. I look different. I feel different. I wear smaller jeans. I even had to put two more notches in my belt.

I continue to run half-marathons. They keep me motivated because I always want to finish. And they're fun. Races are like a festival.

Yeah, I'm hooked on running. I have more energy. I'm more creative, more excited. I go out first thing in the morning when it's quiet and most people are still cozy in bed or sipping their first cup of coffee. Maybe I'll see another runner on the road, and we'll acknowledge each other. It's like being in a secret club. And this is one club I hope to belong to for a very long time.

*Not her real name

in your body's energy bank. Your physical goal is to move your body forward at whatever pace and distance you have set your sights on. Spend energy on side-to-side movements or on the muscular work of trying to make up for biomechanical inefficiencies and you have less to move yourself forward.

So, here's what a strong butt gets you:

Healthy Running + Better Performance = Happy Runner

You Can Control Pain with Strength

As I mentioned earlier, when I was a first-year med student, I tore my ACL—big time—playing soccer. Eventually I had surgery, rehabbed, recovered, and became a runner. Fifteen years after blowing up my knee, I noticed pain in and around the joint. Sure enough, it was arthritis.

In my search for a solution, I tried anything and everything. As a sports doc, I knew I wasn't going to be able to cure the arthritis, but there had to be a way to reduce, if not eliminate, the discomfort so I could keep running. One day I saw a notice for a functional strength-training class being held at Asphalt Green, a fitness center in New York City, and I decided to give it a try. The next day—no kidding—my knee felt better. This was a discovery that would change my running life (and will

change yours) forever. As I got into strength training and plyometrics, I learned that when my legs, hips, and glutes were strong, my knee hurt less. Today these knees have seen 32 marathons and 12 Ironman triathlons, and they are still going strong.

By shouldering more of the physical workload, strong muscles support vulnerable joints. When some of the load of running is transferred from your joints to your muscles, pain eases and injury progression slows down. And that's not all. As I touched on earlier, strong muscles make joints more stable. A stable joint is a healthy joint and is much less likely to get injured, ever.

Muscle Loves Massage

I'm a huge believer in the power of massage. And here's why. When you run or do any repetitive activity that asks your muscles to work (even sitting, which requires your hamstrings to contract), your muscles tighten up, and over time that tightness can contribute to injury. Take Achilles tendonitis, for example, which is inflammation of the tendon that connects your calf muscles to your heel. If your calf muscles are tight, they pull on your Achilles tendon, increasing the tension along it, stressing it out, and setting it up for injury. Regular massage relaxes your muscles, relieves tightness in your calf and tension in the tendon, and helps you avoid one of the most dreaded running injuries.

Now, most of you are pretty familiar with the limbering effects of massage on muscle tissue, but I'm going to give you a few more reasons to regularly put your limbs in the hands of a sports massage therapist. Though we have suspected this for a long time, several scientific studies now show that massage eases the intensity of delayed onset muscle soreness, reduces inflammation, and speeds muscle recovery after exercise. Research at McMaster University in Canada specifically found that massage stimulates the production of mitochondria, the microscopic structures in your muscle fibers that convert nutrients into energy. Flexibility, healthy tissue, full range of motion during running, and speedy recovery—what's not to love about massage?

CAN YOU OD ON EXERCISE?

Some researchers and writers would have you think so. They claim that running multiple marathons in your lifetime or competing in annual Ironman triathlons is bad for your health, raising your risk for heart attack, stroke, and possibly even cancer. With 32 marathons and 12 Ironman triathlons under my belt, I guess I am fast approaching the "finish line of life," as one editorial on extreme exercise puts it. Do I think I should cut way back on exercise? No. Should I cross next year's Ironman Lake Placid off my calendar? I don't think so.

You might wonder if my personal interest has influenced my disregard for these extreme-exercise warnings, like the kid who plugs his ears and spouts loud nothings to avoid hearing his mother's stern reprimand. And I get that. I love endurance exercise and want to keep doing it. But as a physician, I look at the best science and follow the strongest evidence.

These recent studies claiming that loads of endurance exercise will harm your health and shorten your life are small and conflicting. There aren't any big studies showing that marathoners and triathletes are dying young or that longevity declines as the amount of exercise increases. But there is significant evidence that the more physically active you are, the healthier you are and the longer you will live. In Sweden, a review of the medical records of nearly 50,000 men and women who compete in Nordic skiing races of up to 55 miles found that those who completed more races had lowered their risk of death.[1]

And here in the United States, a study of 650,000 individuals showed no decrease in longevity or mortality among those who exercised up to *four times* the minimum recommendation of 30 minutes five times a week.[2] Do the math: Four times the minimum is 2 hours of exercise five times a week. Add to that the tons of studies showing the benefits of regular physical exercise for preventing cardiovascular disease, diabetes, cancer, Alzheimer's, and depression and for improving quality of life—more energy, better daily living, greater happiness, a vibrant mind. So I'm feeling good about sticking to my running schedule, and I hope you are too.

See you on the road—maybe even at Lake Placid.

1. Farahmand, B. Y., A. Ahlbom, O. Ekblom, B. Ekblom, U. Hållmarker, D. Aronson, and G. P. Brobert, "Mortality amongst Participants in Vasaloppet: A Classical Long-Distance Ski Race in Sweden," *Journal of Internal Medicine* 253, no. 3 (March 2003): 276–83.
2. Moore, S. C., A. V. Patel, C. E. Matthews, A. Berrington de Gonzalez, Y. Park, H. A. Katki, M. S. Linet, et al., "Leisure Time Physical Activity of Moderate to Vigorous Intensity and Mortality: A Large Pooled Cohort Analysis," *PLOS Medicine* 9, no. 11 (2012).

Sleep Is the Most Important Activity of the Day

So why do so many of us scrimp on sleep just like we do exercise? It's that too-much-to-do syndrome we seem to be infected with. An ever-increasing number of studies show how important sleep is to the health of our minds and bodies: to memory, focus, cognition, mood, creativity, healthy blood pressure, healthy weight, a healthy immune system. And catching all the z's you need every night makes you a stronger runner. On the flip side, research shows that exercise helps you fall asleep faster, stay asleep longer, and enjoy quality z's, with one caveat, according to the National Sleep Foundation—that you exercise at least 3 hours prior to hitting the pillow.

When you fall asleep, though it's lights out for your conscious self, several other systems are up taking the night shift. These are the hours when your body repairs muscle, builds bone, ramps up red blood cell production, restocks glycogen, and reviews and stores the neuromuscular learning that occurred during your day's run. Cut the shift short and your body doesn't have time to do those jobs thoroughly. Night after night of not enough sleep increasingly wears you down mentally and physically. Not only will your running performance suffer, but you will also be more prone to injury—and, oh yeah, your general health will suffer too.

Earlier I talked about holding daily exercise sacred. Do the same for a good night's sleep. We will talk more about how to get quality rest every night in Chapter 12, but for now take away this: A solid 8 hours makes for great recovery, ensures all systems are ready to go, and puts a shine on your health and a smile on your face. Sweet dreams.

Running Should Be Fun

Hey, I take all of this very seriously and you should too. Running for your health is important stuff, and running competitively can be serious business. But if you don't enjoy it, you won't stick with it. And if it isn't fun, it won't be good for your health. It will be another stress that drags on your mind and beats up your body. Make it happy. Go with friends. Join a running team. Find interesting places to run—city parks, trails, country lanes, historic neighborhoods, river paths. Switch workouts regularly—long runs, short runs, easy runs, hard runs; it keeps things interesting. Race. Whether you make it competitive and run strategically or keep it simple and enjoy the scenery and the company, a race is a great time. It can be a moving party on the road.

Running is complex on a muscular and a molecular level, but it's simple to do: just you, the road, and maybe a friend or a few. You can make it as hard or easy as you want on any given day. It will energize your body and your brain, and it can be the best part of your day.

FOLLOW MY RX FOR HEALTHY RUNNING

So there is the *thinking* behind what's going to help you run your best for the rest of your life, and then there's the *action* you need to take. Here is my prescription for healthy, injury-free running, the details of which you will learn later in this book. Take it and I promise you will build a healthy body, feel great, and get to the finish line faster.

1. **Train for your level of fitness and your goals.**

   Don't run more miles or harder miles than your body can handle.

   Not every runner needs a formal training schedule. If you run for fitness and your goal is 30 minutes a day, that's cool, but if you are just starting out, you need to get there gradually.

2. **Wear the right shoes for your feet and use inserts if you need them.**

   You will hear, if you haven't already, lots of opinions about whether running shoes really help prevent injury and whether you should even wear them. I'm in the camp that thinks the right running shoes can help correct foot-motion issues that lead to injury, and I believe that some of you may need a little added assistance from inserts.

3. **Do the IronStrength workout one or two times a week, every week.**

   If you are one of those runners who has never stepped inside a gym other than to use the treadmill or who hasn't done a pushup since high school fitness testing, get ready to bust some strength moves.

4. **Foam-roll all your muscles every day.**

   You have probably seen them: high-density foam cylinders about 6 inches in diameter that generally come in lengths of 18 or 36 inches. Get one. Get to know it. It will be your body's best friend.

5. **Get 7 to 8 hours of sleep every night.**

   Maybe 6 hours is all you need or 9 is your ideal. But be honest about how much sleep you need and stick to it. Don't get all caught up in the puffery around the water cooler about how much everyone is doing on 5 hours of shut-eye. The cool runner is the one who wins the race and the promotion. Sleep will get you there.

6. **Fuel your body right for running and recovery.**

   A good prerun meal plan is one that keeps you stepping strong. And after a workout or race, you need to deliver the right nutrients to all the microscopic body rebuilders in your muscles so they can do their job and get you back into tip-top shape for your run tomorrow.

7. **Make time (and a budget) for massage twice a month.**

    Your body will thank you. Regular massage is an investment in healthy muscles, faster recovery, and postworkout pain relief. Believe me, it's worth every penny.

8. **Pay attention to pain.**

    I know runners. I have seen plenty of you as patients. You don't quit until you are hobbling around like a lame horse. But by that time, your injury may have progressed to the point of no return to the road for weeks. Here's my rule: When pain changes the way you run, stop running, figure out what's going on, and treat it, and use dynamic rest to stay in shape until you are back on your running feet.

9. **Have fun.**

    Isn't that why we do this?

CHAPTER 2
THE MECHANICS of HEALTHY RUNNING

Running is simple, right? Just push off one foot after the other a bazillion times down the road until you decide to stop or you are too exhausted to take another step. Yep, it's that simple, and that is one of the reasons we love it. But even the simplest things aren't necessarily simplistic.

Lots of neuromuscular connections need to fire for you to pick up your leg, extend it in front of you, plant your foot, push off the ground, and propel your body forward as you run. Here's a quick quiz: Other than chickens (okay, all birds) and humans, what other creatures in the animal kingdom move on two legs? None, right? Even chimps use their arms to scoot across the ground. And why is that? Because two-legged running is really hard. Think Newtonian physics: Gravity wants to take you down, and it's a powerful force to contend with when you are balancing yourself and all your movement on two legs. And when it comes to running, you balance all your body weight on one leg at a time.

There's another g-force that you have to contend with as a runner, and that is ground reaction force (GRF). It's the force coming back at you from the ground as you land. Our friend Newton wrote that every action has an equal and opposite reaction. You strike the ground with a force two to four times your body weight, and the ground strikes back. How your body manages GRF as it enters your foot and travels up your leg has a significant impact on your risk for injury. Big picture—running is simple. Up close—it's pretty complex.

The more you know about how your body works, the better you will be able to understand why injuries happen and how to strengthen your body to prevent them. Bonus: A body built for injury-free running is also prepared to deliver your best performances.

A RUNNER'S MINI DICTIONARY: MUSCLES AND OTHER SOFT STUFF

Fascia: A weblike layer of fibrous connective tissue that covers and wraps around or between muscles, blood vessels, and nerves. It basically keeps all the stuff inside you in its place.

Joint cartilage: Tough but flexible tissue that covers the ends of your bones. It allows smooth movement of your joints and prevents your bones from rubbing against each other.

Ligament: A band of fibrous tissue that connects bone to bone.

Muscle: A band or bundle of fibrous tissue that has the ability to contract, producing movement or maintaining the position of a part of the body.

Tendon: A strong, fibrous band of tissue that connects muscle to bone.

BIG PICTURE: ANATOMY OF A RUNNING STRIDE

Your stride, or gait cycle, begins when one foot touches down on the ground and ends when that same foot hits the ground again. There are two phases: the stance phase, when your foot is in contact with the ground, and the swing phase, when that same foot swings back and then forward before landing again. Here is one complete gait cycle.

1. Your foot makes initial contact with the ground.

2. Your body rolls over your foot while it is planted on the ground (midstance).

3. You toe off or push off the ground.

4. Your leg swings behind you and then forward (swing phase).

5. Your foot strikes the ground again to begin the next gait cycle.

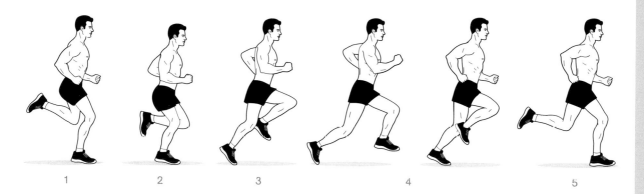

1   2   3   4   5

YOUR BIOMECHANICS FROM FOOT TO HEAD

Your foot has lots of moving parts— 26 bones, 33 joints, 107 ligaments, and 19 muscles and tendons—and for good reason: You need mobility in your foot to cushion impact and to help propel your body forward at toe-off. Foot motion during running goes like this: You land on the outside of your foot (supinate); then, as your weight loads onto your foot, your arch flattens and your foot rolls inward (pronation); then your weight shifts onto the front of your foot toward your big toe, and you push off.

Rolling feet and flattening arches may sound like agents of injury, but trust me, pronation is a good thing; it's normal and necessary for injury prevention.

As your arch flattens, GRF is better absorbed and spread out across your foot. If your arch doesn't flex, your foot remains stiff, and more GRF shoots straight up your shin, putting greater stress on your bone and increasing your chance of a stress injury or, worse, a stress fracture. This lack of motion is called underpronation or oversupination.

You can also overpronate, or have too much motion. This means your foot rolls too far inward before you push off, which puts more strain on the inner side of your shin, which can pull your knee a little out of alignment, increasing your vulnerability to shin and knee trouble.

Whether you overpronate or underpronate or pronate just right indeed depends on your foot structure. If you have a high, rigid arch, you will likely underpronate; if you have a flat foot, you will have a tendency to overpronate. But here's the rub: Foot motion is also influenced by what's happening farther up your body. Let's say there is a lack of stability around your left knee, and as you land, that knee, instead of staying straight ahead, collapses in toward your right knee. When your knee moves inward, it drags your lower leg along; when your lower leg leans in, it encourages your foot to roll further; when your foot rolls too far, you get overpronation; and when you overpronate, you are at greater risk for injuries—among them Achilles tendonitis, stress injuries to the shin, and knee trouble. That is why I'm such a stickler about the strength of your kinetic chain. The stronger the chain, the better you are able to control your body position from above and to dissipate GRF. Plus—I know what you all care about—you'll run faster too!

What I have just described is a series of events along your kinetic chain. Every part of your body has a job to do as you run.

- Your foot is your landing gear. It supports your entire body, but it also works as a lever and helps to propel you forward when you push off.

A RUNNER'S MINI DICTIONARY: STEPS AND STRIDES

Step: A step is counted each time one foot strikes the ground.

Stride: A stride begins when one foot strikes the ground and ends when that same foot strikes the ground again. Two steps (right, left) make one stride. One complete gait cycle is equivalent to one complete stride.

- Then there's your ankle—literally and figuratively overshadowed among joints by the more prominent knee, but it has a ton of responsibility. It's next in line to your foot to absorb GRF, and if it doesn't have a decent amount of flexibility, those forces are headed straight up your leg. Your ankle has a huge motion role to play: It allows movement of your lower leg (followed by the rest of your body) over your foot and facilitates foot motion as you push off. Finally, if the ligaments and muscles around your ankle aren't working for stability, you will be headed for a sprain or a spill. So let's give this joint the respect it deserves.

- Next up, your lower leg, puppeteer to your foot; both upward and downward motion of your foot are controlled by the tibialis anterior in the front teaming up with calf muscles at the back. Lending power to propulsion, your calf muscles also help drive your body forward during toe-off.

- Now to the joint that causes the misinformed to malign running—the knee. (I'm sure someone at some point has told you that running is going to ruin your knees. You can look those people right in the face and tell 'em, "Not true.") Its movement is critical to shock absorption and propulsion. As your knee flexes during footstrike, it reduces GRF, and as you go to push off, extension of your knee produces propulsive force. Stability at this joint is crucial, which is why your knees love your quads.

- The quadriceps—the muscles in the front of your thigh—keep your knee from collapsing as you hit the ground and prevent its rotation during the stance phase of running and as you get ready to push off. (Now you're a big fan too, right?)

- Your hamstrings—at the back of your thigh—don't take a backseat in the action. They partner with your glutes to move your thigh forward during the second half of the swing phase before your foot strikes the ground. They also deliver powerful propulsive force when you push off.

- Your glutes are a gregarious bunch. They like your hammys, but they also hook up with other muscles in your hips and your core to control motion in your pelvis. Rock-solid stability is their signature performance.

- And your arms? While they don't have close contact with the ground (hopefully), they counterbalance what your legs are doing and can help make you a more efficient runner.

While every part of your body has a main job or two to do, all your muscles are working all the time as you run, and they are working

Fun Foot Fact

When you walk or run, as your heel lifts off the ground, your toes are forced to support one-half your body weight.

STEP INTO MY OFFICE

Blipp this page to view a video about the kinetic chain.

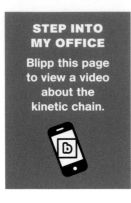

together, not independently. To prevent injury and run your best, you must treat your body as a whole in which the parts are connected and work together in fluid running movement. This is the kinetic chain.

THE BIG K

Kinetic means "relating to motion."

A chain is, of course, a continuous linking of individual parts.

Therefore, a kinetic chain is a chain in motion.

Your running body is a kinetic chain: bones connected to tendons, connected to muscles, connected to tendons, linking joints, and so on from foot to head, all moving in fluid, seamless motion. When all the pieces are healthy and strong, the entire chain is strong, work is distributed evenly, everybody's happy, and performance is great. But if one piece of the chain is weak, another has to make up for that weakness and take on more of the workload. Over time, the extra burden can wear down the load bearer; it becomes overly stressed and hurt, and it may call in sick the next time you decide to go for a run.

Here's a scenario I have seen play out with some of my patients. As you know, your glutes and hamstrings work together to bring your thigh up in front of you, control your leg during footstrike, and propel you off the ground at push-off. If you have a weak butt, more of that work gets pushed onto your hamstrings. Day after day, that extra workload stresses out your hammys and they start to hurt. Eventually, the stress may even cause a tear.

THREE SIMPLE STEPS TO AN AWESOME KINETIC CHAIN

So, how do you get a great kinetic chain and improve your running mechanics? Here are the steps. For all the details, turn to Chapter 12.

1. Strengthen your whole body twice a week. Certain muscles get a great workout when you run; others more or less come along for the ride. If running is your only activity, you have strength imbalances. Total-body functional strength training twice a week with my IronStrength workout will fix that and help you maintain a strong balance.

2. Work on flexibility every day. If you don't already have a foam roller, I want you to get one. Use it every day to loosen tight spots and to maintain flexibility in all your muscles.

3. Rest. Get enough sleep, yes, but I also want you to build dynamic rest into your training. Don't go all out every day. Follow hard training with easy training to allow your body to recoup and regroup. Remember that rest is a powerful agent for building strength.

THE AT-HOME TEST FOR RUNNING IMBALANCE

If you have an injury-threatening imbalance, you will likely find it in your hip abductors. These often-ignored muscles on the outside of the hip work at keeping your hips stable. If you have a weakness on one side, that hip will drop as you run, creating extra motion at your knee.

To test yourself at home, stand in front of a mirror and do single-leg squats, first on one side and then the other. Smooth and steady motion on each leg means you are strong right and left. If you wobble on one side, it shows you that your muscles are weaker on that side; also, you won't be able to squat as low on that side.

The other test I like to use is the step-down. Get an 18- to 24-inch-high stool or wooden box and set it in front of a mirror. Stand on it and step down slowly once from each side. As you step down, watch your pelvic bone; if one side drops as you lower down to the floor, you have a muscular imbalance on that side and need to do some strength work. Single-leg squats, side planks, and bridges are good for hips, butt, and core.

You can make do-it-yourself testing more fun and more informative with an app such as Ubersense, Coach's Eye, or Dartfish. Download any of these to your smartphone or tablet and videotape yourself doing single-leg squats and step-downs, or get a friend to tape you, and then play it back in slow motion or look at individual frames of your movement. You can even create lines across your pictured form to help you see how your body parts line up at different phases of movement.

Workload imbalance between side-by-side coworkers isn't the only cause of stress in the system. A weak link can create kinks in your chain that put extra stress on areas elsewhere. Here's another scenario—and one that I see all the time. The muscles in your hip, butt, and core form the stability-central group. They work together to hold you steady as you run. Weakness in one or more of those muscles allows your pelvis to drop. When your pelvis drops, your knee collapses inward; when your knee collapses inward, your foot rolls too far to the inside. Maybe you will be fortunate enough to have high-functioning quads that keep your knee in line, but maybe not—and then you become vulnerable to injuries of the shin, knee, and hip.

Keep in mind, too, that trouble doesn't always travel in one direction. Sore shins may result from weakness up in stability central; they may also be caused by poor footwork. If you get injured, search up and down your kinetic chain for the cause.

Lastly, it's not always weak muscles that lead to injury. Tight muscles create trouble in the chain too. Tight calves, for example, pull on your Achilles tendon, creating tension that may eventually turn into tendonitis. Your hamstrings attach to the top of your pelvis, and if they are too tight, they will pull your pelvis down, which strains muscles in your lower back. Keeping muscles flexible can help prevent pain and injury.

WHY WE GET HURT

Okay, so you've got this complex kinetic chain of muscles, tendons, bones, ligaments, and joints, and when a piece of the chain is too weak or too tight, it makes you vulnerable to injury when you run. But still, there's no bike to crash, no opponent to battle; no one is going to tackle you to the ground or slam into you to stop you from running. There's no twisting, swinging, jumping. You're just moving straight ahead, a few inches off the ground. So why the heck do runners get injured? That's a great question, and here are the answers.

Because running is one foot after the other for miles and miles. If you have a tight calf that is pulling on your Achilles tendon, a lap or two around the block isn't going to tear your tendon, but miles of running every day plus 20-milers on the weekend, combined with a continued lack of flexibility, will eventually traumatize that tendon, and you will be off the road nursing Achilles tendonitis. Running is repetitive. Keep hammering a weak link and eventually it breaks. This is the madness that causes an overuse injury. The solution, which we will talk about in detail later, is not only to address the weakness but also to include periods of rest in your training that allow your body to rebuild and restore itself in readiness for your next run.

Because you have succumbed to doing too much too soon. Let's say that, for whatever reason, you haven't been able to run in several months, and, in fact, you have been a couch potato all that time, so you have lost aerobic conditioning, mus-

STRIDE RIGHT

While I don't recommend that you spend a lot of time fixing your form, if you are a heel-striker, I do want you to work toward landing on your midfoot. Here's why.

1. With a midfoot strike, you have more bend at your knee and your leg lands closer to your body rather than straight out in front of you. This improves shock absorption and reduces the stress to your knees, hips, and back.

2. When you land on your midfoot rather than on your heel, your foot spends less time on the ground, which increases your running efficiency and may translate into faster running times.

   Shoot for your right or left leg to hit the ground 85 to 90 times per minute. It might feel weird when you first start shortening your stride, but I have found, both as a runner and a doc, that it does wonders for all aspects of running health.

cle strength, and bone strength. But now you are eager to get back on the road, and as an experienced runner, you figure you can start logging weekly miles almost as if you had never stopped.

Scenario 2: You have been following a steady diet of 25 miles a week, but then a friend convinces you to enter a marathon that is only 2 months away. Your longest run is a 5-miler, so you pile the miles into your weekly log and on top of your weekly long run.

Scenario 3: You're a marathoner and you just completed your eighth 26.2-miler. You're itching to try something new, so you decide to jump into a mile race on the track without training for it. You ask your long, slow-distance muscles to find a short, fast gear.

In each of these scenarios, you put your body under a lot of stress because you are asking it to do something it hasn't done before (run fast when you have only run slow miles) or isn't accustomed to (run lots of miles when you have been logging low or no miles). Stress is a good thing in the right dose. You need to stress your body in new ways to build strength and speed and to train your neuro-muscular pathways to perform well and efficiently for the work you want to do. But you've got to do it gradually. You have to teach your body new moves and give it time to learn and develop bone strength and muscle strength. Dump a heavy load on a limb that's not prepared to take it, and it will get hurt.

Because you are out of line. When the wheels of your car are out of alignment, the tires wear unevenly, steering becomes screwy, braking becomes uneven, and the suspension is compromised, which leads to rough riding and more wear and tear. This isn't so different than what happens when your body is out of alignment, or imbalanced.

When I see runners who generally seem pretty healthy—no significant or obvious structural issues—and who follow a levelheaded training plan but have a problem with injury, I will send them to our running clinic at the Hospital for Special Surgery, where one of our great physical therapists, like Michael Silverman, will perform a running analysis to try to figure out what's going on. If you were to visit with Michael, he would first check your muscle strength, flexibility and range of motion, and posture. He then tests for dynamic stability—measuring how stable or wobbly you are as you do single-leg squats and step-downs. And finally, he films and analyzes a video of you running on a treadmill. All of this makes up your running mechanics profile. (It's way cool.) Here are the 10 points of a perfect profile.

1. **Good muscle strength and endurance.** Strength is the force your muscle exerts; endurance is how long your muscle can continue to exert that force. You need balanced strength and endurance throughout your body to run your best and sidestep injury. Think back to the kinetic chain: A weak or fatigued muscle throws off the balance by shifting more work onto other parts of the chain.

2. **Not too little or too much flexibility.** You want enough flexibility in your muscles, tendons, ligaments, and other soft tissue to allow full range of motion for optimal performance and injury prevention. Stiff joints don't absorb GRF very well, and a tight muscle pulls on the other links in your chain. But too much flexibility isn't a good thing either. Imagine running with limbs like Slinkys: You would wobble wildly as you ran, forcing your body to work harder for stability and generating new pathways for injury as your limbs fall out of alignment. And when it comes to running performance, your muscles act like springs to propel you up and forward. Some stiffness in the coil creates way more propulsive force than if you had Slinkys for legs. As I always tell my patients, I would much rather you be strong than flexible.

3. **Proper posture.** A healthy spine equals healthy running. Misalignment of your vertebrae causes missteps when you run—less-than-ideal stride length and frequency—and throws off your overall alignment. The most obvious and egregious example is the runner with scoliosis, an abnormal curvature of the

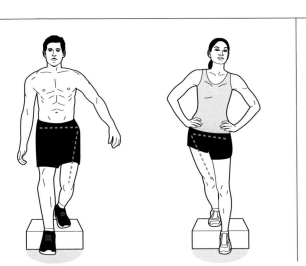 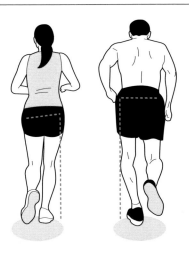

When you do the step-down test or run, ideally your hips will remain horizontal and parallel to the ground as you see in the male runner. If your hip dips on one or both sides (female runner), strengthen your muscle to improve stability.

spine, which can cause a tilt in the hips that then creates a functional leg-length discrepancy: The leg on your raised-hip side will appear and function as a shorter leg. That really shakes up the kinetic chain.

4. **Solid dynamic stability.** When you do a step-down, you want smooth control as you lower down, no flailing and wobbling. And if you were to draw a straight line across your pelvis from left to right, you would want that line to stay parallel to the floor as you step down. If either or both sides drop, it means you are weak on one or both sides of your hips.

5. **A level pelvis when you run.** As with the step-downs, you want to run with a horizontal hip line, parallel to the ground. Too much motion in the ocean rocks your kinetic chain out of alignment.

6. **A short stride with a midfoot strike pattern.** When you run, you want to land on your midfoot with your leg close to your body. This alignment improves absorption of GRF. If you land on your heel with your foot in front of you, your leg will be straighter; you will "brake" harder as you run, which increases GRF up your leg. (See "Stride Right" on page 24 for how to score a short stride and a great landing.)

7. **Feet that pronate just right.** Land, roll, and push off without spending too much time on the outside or inside of your foot. Here's the deal: Your foot is essentially a lever that pries you off the ground and helps push you forward, so it needs some rigidity to do that. But it's also the first part of your body to hit the ground, so it must have flexibility to absorb and buffer GRF. Good foot

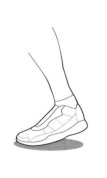
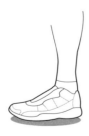
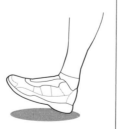

Footstrike patterns (left to right): forefoot, midfoot, heel.

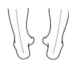

Degree of pronation (top to bottom): underpronation, normal pronation, overpronation.

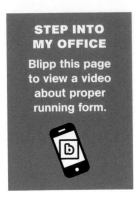

STEP INTO MY OFFICE

Blipp this page to view a video about proper running form.

structure and motion allows both of these. First, you land on the outside of your foot (the supinated position), which is somewhat rigid and helps brake or control your forward motion so you don't fall flat on your face. Next, you roll over your foot (pronation), at which point your flexible arch spreads out to absorb GRF. And finally, you roll forward on your foot toward your big toe (supination), which provides the rigidity you need to push off the ground. Rigid, soft, rigid.

8. **A 5- to 7-centimeter liftoff.** Too much up and down movement is a waste of your time and energy. The good news is that as you run and as you develop a shorter stride, you will naturally fall into the best range of motion.

9. **Straight up and down at mid-stance.** When your foot is fully planted on the ground, you should be able to drop a plumb line straight down from hip to foot, perpendicular to the ground. Again, this alignment is optimal for shock absorption.

10. **Arms that swing alternately from front to back.** Coaches and sports specialists offer up a variety of opinions about how you should use your arms while you run, but there is little research other than studies showing that you're better off letting them swing naturally forward and back than you are running with your hands clasped behind your head, crossed in front of your chest, or held behind your back. What we know for sure is that arm

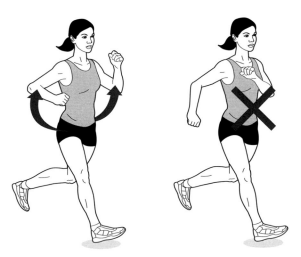

As you run, your arms should swing forward and backward, not across your body.

movement counterbalances leg movement. As your right leg moves forward, so does your left arm. It's all about balance and stability, and you know how much I love stability. If you were to run with your hands on your head, your torso would be twisting all over the place to balance out leg motion. There is also some debate as to whether it really matters if your arms swing across your chest, but I'm in the camp that believes a simple, relaxed forward and backward arm swing is most efficient and gets you the best results.

So do you need a perfect mechanical profile (aka form) to run well and healthy? No. Emil Zatopek—the gold medal winner of the 5,000 meters, 10,000 meters, and marathon at the 1952 Olympic Games who was named the Greatest Runner of All Time by

Runner's World magazine—ran with a peculiar side-to-side roll of his head and an occasional tilt to his torso. If you don't get injured and are comfortable with the way you are, I say stick with it. You are what you are. Your genes and individual biomechanics will, to a large extent, determine your form, but that doesn't mean you can't tweak it. Running is straight-ahead, linear motion. No juking, no jumping, no turning, no twisting. To run your best and your healthiest, you want good vertical alignment from heel to head and strong horizontal stability across your hips. Knees that wobble, hips that dip, feet that flop too much or too little—these are signs of weakness and imbalance that rock your kinetic chain. But I have great news for you, which I know firsthand as a runner and triathlete: No matter what your age or ability, you can fix and finesse your kinetic chain to run better and healthier than ever.

PART II

Uh-Oh: What's That Pain?

You went out for a run and felt a pain in your leg, but you just kept running. The next day, you ran again and that same pain hurt a little more. You have a big race coming, though, so you toughed it out again and again the next day, but the pain keeps getting worse. What the heck is going on? Let's find out.

CHAPTER 3

ACHES and PAINS from the FEET UP

The best-laid plans, right? Injuries happen, even when you're running smart.

Welcome to my virtual doctor's office.

I'm going to take you through the same steps I follow when I see patients in my real-life office at the Hospital for Special Surgery in New York City.

1. We will look at where it hurts and figure out what's going on.

2. I will tell you how to treat it at home and when you need to see a doctor.

3. I will explain how you can prevent the injury from happening again.

Now, here's the really cool part. Along with the printed advice in the pages ahead, you will be able to use the free app to scan pages to link you to videos filmed in my office, where, with the help of Rex the skeleton and real-life runner Meghan, I will show you exactly where injuries occur as I explain what's going on and what to do. You are literally walking into my office with your smartphone from wherever you are around the world! For some of you, like my Aussie friends, this is a *really* long-distance consultation.

And there's more—a virtual gym! I have filmed demonstrations of the exercises you need to do to get healthy and keep running. Not only will you learn to diagnose yourself, you will also learn to fix and prevent your aches and pains at home.

When I said welcome to my virtual office, I meant it.

But before we jump into the specifics of the aches and pains you have now or might get, I want to answer a few common questions I get from runners—questions that you might have too.

Is It Soreness or Something More Serious?

Runners come into my office all the time saying, "Doc, I felt this pain in my [foot/shin/hip/whatever]—but it really wasn't that bad at first, so I kept running. And I tried a few stretches that my running partner suggested, but that didn't help. The pain got worse, and now I can't run at all."

There's injury prevention, and then there's preventing a mild injury from becoming a major one. The key is to recognize when soreness or mild pain is a sign that something more serious will happen if you don't take care of it. My general rule here is that a little bit of pain is okay, but pain that changes the way you move needs to be checked out. For example, if your shin aches a bit when you run, that's probably okay, but shin pain that changes the way you run definitely needs a diagnosis and both a treatment and a prevention plan.

If Inflammation Is the Body's Natural Response to Injury, Why Are We Always Trying to Get Rid of It?

This is a tough one. Inflammation is both a blessing and a curse. In the short term, when you strain, say, a muscle, inflammation is responsible for the recruitment of specialized cells to that tissue to promote healing. Chronic inflammation, however, is a different story. A chronically inflamed Achilles

DOCTOR WHO?

When it's time to see a doc about a running injury, look for a sports medicine physician. This is an MD who has additional specific training in diagnosing, treating, and preventing sports injuries. And if you can, find one who participates in sports—a sports doc who is also a runner ideally. Not only will that doctor have the added knowledge that comes with personal experience, but she will understand your love of the sport and will be committed to getting you back on the road.

tendon, for example, can start to actually degenerate over time. Tendonitis (acute inflammation) can lead to tendonosis (chronic inflammation), which can lead to a tear in the tendon.

So what's a runner to do?

Ice—nature's anti-inflammatory. It's safe, it works, and it helps prevent acute inflammation from becoming chronic.

Why Am I in More Pain 2 Days after a Hard Run Than I Was 2 Hours after That Run?

Four words: delayed onset muscle soreness, or DOMS. Anytime you ask your muscles to work harder than they are accustomed to, that extra strain does a little damage, breaking some of the muscle fibers. This is actually a good thing because when your body repairs that damage, it builds a stronger muscle. It's the same response you get when you strength-train. But back to DOMS. For years experts blamed the buildup of lactic acid for the pain, but that theory has been debunked. DOMS is the product of complex physiological processes that take place within the muscle after intense exercise. Special cells, along with an array of enzymes and other chemicals, are coming and going, cleaning up dead tissue, removing waste products, and constructing new tissue. All this cellular activity causes pain. The big picture looks like this.

1. A hard workout causes muscle trauma.

2. Some soreness occurs afterward in response to the trauma.

3. Twelve to 24 hours after your run, rebuilding begins and soreness increases.

4. Soreness disappears after a couple of days.

5. Muscles are stronger.

6. Performance is improved.

If you are new to running, you may be experiencing DOMS right now. Trust me, your muscles will adapt and you will be able to run pain-free. But even experienced runners get DOMS after an intense-speed workout or race, after a marathon, or after a grueling hill workout.

If you haven't already, you are going to experience DOMS, whether it's from increases in training or from beginning my IronStrength workouts (strengthening your muscles, by the way, helps prevent and relieve DOMS). You can minimize it by not overdoing it. Plan gradual increases in mileage, speed work, and hill training, and make sure you drink plenty of fluids regularly. When you feel the soreness that comes with a new or hard workout or a race, just go with it, knowing it means your body is busy repairing and rebuilding stronger. You will be a better athlete for it.

STEP INTO MY OFFICE

Blipp this page to view a video addressing common questions patients often ask Dr. Metzl.

Would I Ever Need to See a Doc about DOMS?

In 99 percent of cases, there is no need to see a doctor about delayed onset muscle soreness. It resolves on its own. But if you experience severe muscle soreness and your urine is dark, see a sports physician. When muscle is injured, it releases a protein called myoglobin. In rare cases of DOMS, a large amount of myoglobin is produced, which can damage kidneys. This is called rhabdomyolysis, and it can cause permanent damage, so beware. Your doctor can run blood and urine tests to check.

What's the Difference between a Strain and a Sprain?

All kinds of words get thrown around when we're talking about injuries. You hear runners say:

I pulled my hamstring.

I have a calf strain.

I sprained my ankle.

I ruptured my Achilles.

But what are we really talking about here? Let's start with sprains and strains, which are similar types of injuries occurring in different kinds of tissue.

A *sprain* is an overstretched or torn ligament. A ligament is a strong band of fibrous tissue that connects bone to bone, which means sprains occur at your joints: ankles, knees, hips, wrists, and so forth.

A *strain* is an overstretched or torn muscle or tendon. Tendons are the strong bands of fibrous tissue that connect muscle to bone and are located near joints (think Achilles tendon). When people say they've *pulled* a muscle, they're referring to a strain—it just sounds more dramatic.

Strains are categorized by severity into three grades. A grade 1 strain

PRP: CUTTING-EDGE TREATMENT

Can't kick an injury? Your doctor might try PRP, which stands for platelet-rich plasma. If a runner has a soft-tissue injury that has been around for 4 to 5 months and isn't healing on its own, I may recommend PRP as a way to recruit the body's own healing potential and inject it at a targeted location that isn't healing. Here's the deal: Blood speeds healing in injured tissue, but with tendons in particular, bloodflow is limited. PRP puts platelets and the more important platelet-derived growth factor (PDF) right where you need them. First, I will do an MRI to examine the injured area. To prepare for the injection, blood is drawn from the patient's arm and then spun down in a centrifuge to concentrate the platelets, blood cells that aid in healing. Then that platelet-rich plasma is injected at the site of the injury. Common sites where I perform PRP on runners include the proximal hamstring (top of your hamstring just below your pelvis), Achilles tendon, and plantar fascia.

BACK ON THE ROAD

The first question you will ask if you get injured will be "What's going on?" immediately followed by "Can I keep running with this pain?" I have two rules for you.

Rule 1: If pain forces you to change the way you run, you need to stop. Continuing to run with altered form can cause further injury along your kinetic chain, and you could be sidelined for a long time. Here's the good news: You can choose an activity you can do without pain, whether that's swimming, cycling, elliptical training, whatever. I call this *dynamic rest*. This way you can keep up your conditioning so that when you do return to running, you can slip back in near the level when you had to stop.

Rule 2: When the day-to-day pain from an injury is gone and you feel ready, go for a test run—a slow run of about 10 minutes. If it hurts, stop running and give it a couple more days before you try again.

means you have overstretched the tendon or muscle and may have torn a small percentage of muscle fibers; pain is mild. Grade 2 strains involve tears in the muscle or tendon. A grade 3 is either a severe tear or your muscle and tendon are torn apart, or *ruptured*. This is a strain to the max. It really hurts, and if you have a complete rupture, you won't be able to use that muscle until the tendon has been repaired, usually surgically.

How Do I Look Up My Injury If I Don't Know What It Is?

Good question. I have tried to make this book as user-friendly as possible. Where's your pain? If it's in your knee, turn to the knee chapter. The following chapters are organized from foot to head. At the beginning of each chapter, I give a brief list of the symptoms you might be experiencing along with the probable injuries. Read through the list, identify the symptoms that most closely resemble yours, and then turn to the corresponding injury for all the gory details. So if the symptoms of that knee pain appear to match those for runner's knee, for example, turn to that injury to learn more.

With each injury, I provide deeper detail about the symptoms, I explain what the injury is and its possible causes, and then I tell you how to fix it and prevent it from hopefully ever happening again. If you're currently healthy, that's terrific. But if you are prone to hip problems, for example, I suggest you turn to those pages to see if you're doing everything you can to stay healthy. You will find strength exercises, stretches, and foam roller moves, as well as videos in which I explain how to do these moves—you can even watch a demonstration. I'll see you in my virtual office!

When Do I Actually Need to See a Doctor?

I have designed this book and filmed the accompanying videos to teach you how to take care of yourself. If what I suggest isn't working, or if you're getting worse, you need to go see a doctor. Even if you're the smartest runner in Brussels, seeing someone with medical training is important if you're not getting better.

CHAPTER 4

YOUR FEET and ANKLES

With each step you take as you run, your body—all of it—lands with a force two to four times your weight on one foot that is, for most of us, not more than 12 inches long and about 4 inches wide.

Your foot is the first piece in your kinetic chain to absorb shock, hold you vertical, and push you off the ground as you run. And that means not only is it vulnerable to injury, but how it does its job is going to be felt all the way up your kinetic chain. If you overpronate (your foot rolls excessively inward), for example, you are at greater risk for foot problems as well as injuries to your Achilles tendons, shins, knees, even your hips. So let's give your feet the respect they deserve.

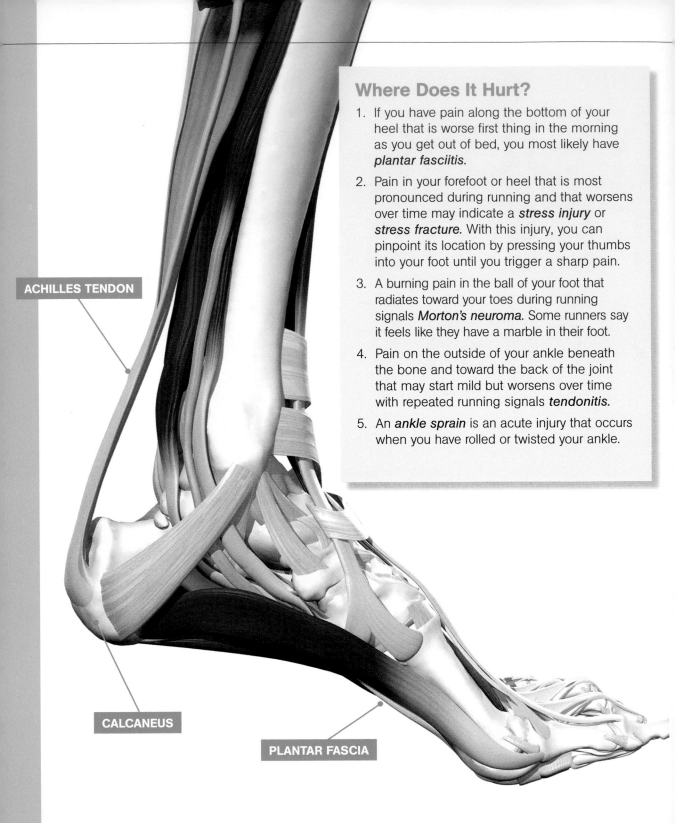

ACHILLES TENDON

CALCANEUS

PLANTAR FASCIA

Where Does It Hurt?

1. If you have pain along the bottom of your heel that is worse first thing in the morning as you get out of bed, you most likely have *plantar fasciitis.*

2. Pain in your forefoot or heel that is most pronounced during running and that worsens over time may indicate a *stress injury* or *stress fracture.* With this injury, you can pinpoint its location by pressing your thumbs into your foot until you trigger a sharp pain.

3. A burning pain in the ball of your foot that radiates toward your toes during running signals *Morton's neuroma.* Some runners say it feels like they have a marble in their foot.

4. Pain on the outside of your ankle beneath the bone and toward the back of the joint that may start mild but worsens over time with repeated running signals *tendonitis.*

5. An *ankle sprain* is an acute injury that occurs when you have rolled or twisted your ankle.

Plantar Fasciitis

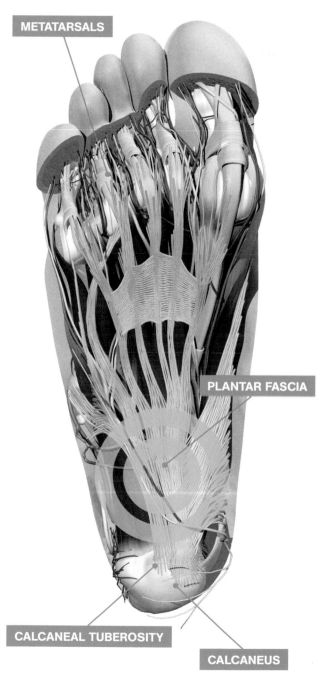

METATARSALS

PLANTAR FASCIA

CALCANEAL TUBEROSITY

CALCANEUS

You have all heard the horror stories of the 3 years of plantar fasciitis. This can be the bane of many runners' lives. One day you're running along smiling at the world, the next day your heel aches and you're miserable. Plantar (referring to the bottom of your foot) fasciitis (inflammation of the fascia, a thin layer of connective tissue that covers muscle) strikes fear in the heart of almost every runner. Even if you have never had it, you likely know someone who has, and you have heard his curses. Please do not take this injury lightly—ignore plantar fasciitis and very quickly it can hobble you with pain and sideline you from running for a long time. I had it once for 7 months, and I never want to have it again.

SYMPTOMS

- You will feel pain in your heel that is worse first thing in the morning. Though the pain is usually located on the inner (medial) side of the heel, you may feel it toward the center of the bottom of your heel or farther up toward the arch.

- During running, the pain limits your ability to push off.

WHAT'S GOING ON?

The plantar fascia is a band of connective tissue that runs from the heel bone, or the calcaneus, along the bottom of your foot to the metatarsals. It helps support your foot's arch and give it shape, and it aids in providing stability as your foot strikes the ground and then pushes off. The fascia stretches as you land and contracts as your foot comes off the ground. Excess tension or pulling of the fascia causes inflammation, usually at the origin of the fascia at the calcaneal tuberosity (the bump on the bottom of your

41

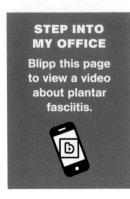

**STEP INTO
MY OFFICE**

**Blipp this page
to view a video
about plantar
fasciitis.**

heel). Left untreated, microtears develop in the inflamed tissue, which leads to debilitating pain.

If you have very high-arched feet, you are more prone to this injury because a high arch creates more tension in the fascia. But what goes on above the foot can also cause trouble. The plantar fascia is part of the tendo-Achilles complex: Your calf muscles hook into the Achilles tendon, which connects to the back of the calcaneus, and off the front of the calcaneus comes the plantar fascia. Tight muscles in the calf pull on the Achilles, which pulls on the calcaneus, which pulls on the plantar fascia. The result: inflammation, tearing of the tissue—and pain.

WHAT TO DO

- Use dynamic rest. Bike, swim, use an elliptical trainer, run in the pool—whatever activity you can do pain-free as you treat the inflammation and figure out why it happened.

- Chill your foot in a bucket of ice water, or freeze water in a paper cup and roll your foot over it.

- Take an anti-inflammatory, such as ibuprofen or naproxen, to help reduce inflammation and pain.

- Pump your ankle up and down 10 to 15 times every day before getting out of bed. This helps loosen up the Achilles tendon and fascia before you load it with pressure when you stand.

- Keep a pair of shoes, sandals, or slippers with good arch support next to your bed and slip into them first thing in the morning. The fascia will have tightened up overnight, and a shoe with arch support will reduce tension to the tissue and prevent pain.

- During the day, try to loosen the plantar fascia by rolling the middle of your arch over a golf or tennis ball, but don't roll the ball over the bone where it hurts. This reduces the tension pulling on the site of pain.

- Stretch your calf muscles—using the basic calf stretches at the end of this chapter—to lessen tension along the tendo-Achilles complex.

- Consider purchasing foot splints to wear while you sleep. A variety of options are widely available. It's best to ask your doctor to recommend one that's right for your case.

- If after 2 weeks of home treatment your pain hasn't improved, make an appointment with a sports doc. In addition to recommending that you continue with the treatments listed here, he may suggest a cortisone injection. If that fails to provide relief, the next step may be platelet-rich plasma (PRP) injections (see "PRP: Cutting-Edge Treatment" on page 36 to learn the details).

PREVENTION

The key to preventing plantar fasciitis is a strong and flexible kinetic chain. Though this is an injury to the foot, it can be caused by what's happening farther up the chain.

- Do the IronStrength workout once or twice a week (see Chapter 12 and watch the videos).

- Strengthen the muscles of your feet with some barefoot running or by running or walking in minimalist shoes.

- Massage and loosen the plantar fascia by rolling your foot over a tennis ball for a few minutes every day.

- Use your foam roller daily to massage your calf muscles as shown at the end of this chapter.

- Perform the simple calf stretches shown at the end of this chapter.

- Try orthotics. Over-the-counter (OTC) arch supports inserted into your running shoes can be helpful, especially if you have high arches. You can also purchase prescription orthotics, custom-made for your foot, but I have found that 90 percent of my patients get good results with OTC ones. I love heat-moldable inserts. Lots of companies make them; search online.

- Check your stride. A shorter stride and quicker cadence may help by reducing the load on your foot. Aim for 170 to 180 footstrikes per minute (counted every time your feet hit the ground).

WHY DOES IT TAKE SO LONG TO RECOVER FROM PLANTAR FASCIITIS?

That's a great question. The body's healing response is proportional to bloodflow, of which there is very little to the plantar fascia. This is why PRP injections speed healing in most runners with this injury. I generally don't recommend PRP unless the pain has been present for more than 4 months and other treatments haven't worked.

Stress Fracture of the Foot

You have an ache in your foot; it hurts a little bit; and then it hurts more. Before you know it, you're limping to work. A stress fracture is a type of overuse injury. This means that unlike an acute traumatic injury, like a concussion, that occurs in an instant, a stress fracture happens from repetitive loading over time. In fact, stress fractures were initially described in military recruits who were marching all day long. It's important to recognize that stress fractures can happen in any bone in the body depending on the sport you're doing. Gymnasts get stress fractures in their wrists, rowers get stress fractures in their ribs, and runners get stress fractures in their feet, shins, and hips.

SYMPTOMS

- Landing on your foot hurts, so you change your running mechanics to ease up on that foot.

- You can pinpoint the source of the pain when you press your fingers into the bone at the area of tenderness. Most stress fractures of the foot occur in the metatarsals—the long, slender bones—but they can also happen in the heel bone (calcaneus) and the tarsal navicular, a bone located at the top of your foot close to your ankle (see the illustration).

- You may or may not have swelling; look to see if the top of your injured foot appears different than your healthy foot.

- Do the single-leg hop test: Try to hop on the suspect foot; if you feel lots of pain when you land on the foot, see your doctor.

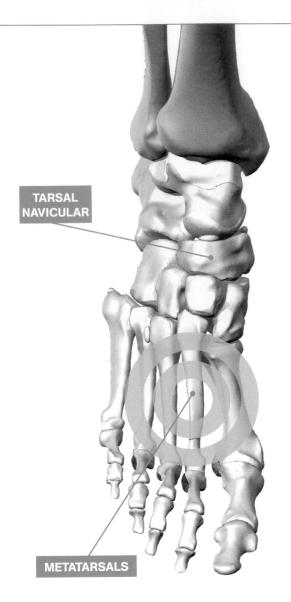

TARSAL NAVICULAR

METATARSALS

STEP INTO MY OFFICE
Blipp this page to view a video about the prevention and treatment of stress fractures.

WHAT'S GOING ON

This is a classic overuse injury. Unlike a broken bone, which results from a traumatic event such as a fall or twist, a stress fracture develops over time due to repetitive loading, as happens with running. The demand on the bone simply exceeds the bone's ability to withstand the force. The bone swells inside—called a stress reaction or stress injury—and with continued loading it can eventually fracture. No two stress fractures are the same. The defining factor is location, location, location. Consider the tarsal navicular bone I mentioned. It gets little bloodflow, and blood is essential to healing. So a stress fracture in this bone is going to take longer to heal and requires a different treatment plan than a stress fracture to a metatarsal.

Three key factors put you at risk for a stress injury or fracture.

1. Increasing your mileage too quickly. Bone adapts to the loading force of running, but it needs time to get stronger in response to that force.

2. Poor running mechanics: overpronation or overstriding. Also, weak core and hip muscles can lead to sloppy running mechanics.

3. Low bone density (osteopenia) or very low bone density (osteoporosis), which leaves bones brittle. Causes include genetics; low calcium intake; and, for women, amenorrhea (missing three or more menstrual cycles in a row), which lowers the amount of circulating estrogen, important to bone health. All of us acquire 90 percent of our lifetime bone density by age 18, and women reach their maximum bone density by age 32. After that, maintenance is essential.

STEP INTO MY OFFICE

Blipp this page to view a video about treatment of injuries sustained through overuse.

WHAT TO DO

- If you suspect a stress fracture, see a sports doctor ASAP. Taking care of this injury right away can be the difference between 4 weeks and 4 months of recovery. Your doc will order an x-ray or MRI. Typically stress fractures don't show up on x-rays unless they are well on their way to cracking (very serious) or already in the healing stage, during which the body makes a callus—a bump on the bone at the site of the injury.

- If the tests come back confirming a stress fracture, your doctor may also request a bone density scan, depending on your case and family history, to try to figure out why the injury happened.

- Work with your doctor to understand the cause of your injury and plan a strategy that will help you heal and prevent a recurrence.

- If you overpronate, try over-the-counter arch supports. I like heat-moldable orthotics, which you can find online. If they don't work and you continue to get stress fractures, consider custom orthotics.

- If your diet is low in calcium, eat more calcium- and vitamin D–rich foods. Dairy products are the best sources (see Chapter 15 for other options).

- Use dynamic rest to maintain fitness (swimming is a great option), but avoid activities that put weight on your injured foot, and continue with upper-body strength training.

- Before you attempt running again, consult with your doctor. Any running on a stress fracture that hasn't healed can reverse the gains you have made toward recovery.

PREVENTION

- Follow the 10 percent rule—don't up your mileage by more than 10 percent a week.

- If you overpronate, choose shoes that limit pronation. Arch supports can help as well.

- Make sure you get enough calcium and vitamin D daily: 1,000 milligrams of calcium (women over 50 and men over 70 should take 1,200 milligrams); 600 IU of vitamin D (all adults over 70 should take 800 IU). The best sources are dairy products (see Chapter 15 for other options).

- Strengthen your core and hips by doing the IronStrength workout once or twice a week (see Chapter 12 and watch the videos). Strengthening these areas will improve your running mechanics.

- Try shortening your stride. A shorter stride and faster foot cadence reduces stress to your lower legs. Count every time your feet hit the ground for 1 minute—aim for 170 to 180 footstrikes.

Morton's Neuroma

This foot injury is 8 to 10 times more common in women than men. The reason? If you guessed the willingness among many (but not all, of course) women to sacrifice comfort for fashion, you are correct. High heels and other shoes that squeeze the forefoot are the number-one cause of Morton's neuroma—the result of an angry nerve that has had to endure being squished.

SYMPTOMS

- You will experience a burning pain in the ball of your foot that radiates toward your toes during running.

- You may feel tingling or numbness between your third and fourth toes.

- As the injury worsens, you may feel pain during walking or even at rest.

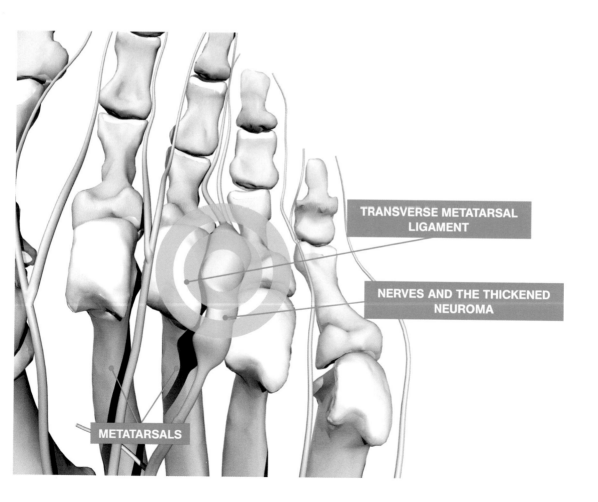

TRANSVERSE METATARSAL LIGAMENT

NERVES AND THE THICKENED NEUROMA

METATARSALS

WHAT'S GOING ON

Morton's neuroma is a thickening of one of the nerves in your foot (the plantar digital nerve) where it passes beneath the transverse metatarsal ligament (see illustration on page 47).

When your forefoot is constricted by tight shoes, for example, the nerve gets squeezed up against the ligament, and repeated rubbing against that ligament causes inflammation and enlargement.

WHAT TO DO

- If the pain causes you to change the way you run, switch to an activity that you can do pain-free and continue with upper-body strength training.

- Try an anti-inflammatory, such as ibuprofen or naproxen, to relieve inflammation.

- Switch your running and everyday shoes to pairs with a wider toe box and good arch support to help relieve pressure.

- Try over-the-counter shoe inserts (I like heat-moldable orthotics, which you can find online), which may help relieve pressure on the irritated nerve. If they don't provide relief, consider custom orthotics.

- If pain persists despite home treatments, see a sports doc, who may recommend a cortisone injection to shrink the neuroma. When cortisone injections fail to relieve the pain, surgery is the next option—but it should be considered a last resort since it might create forefoot instability, which can lead to further problems down the road.

PREVENTION

- Choose your footwear wisely. Shoes, running or otherwise, should be snug while allowing your toes some wiggle room (see Chapter 16 for details on how to get the right fit).

- Women who wear shoes that constrict the forefoot should keep it to a minimum. Kick off your heels as soon as you can and slip your feet into something comfy.

Ankle Tendonitis (aka Peroneal Tendonitis)

You don't want to mess with injuries to tendons. Ignore an inflamed tendon and it gets really angry—it swells up and may even tear. To make matters worse, there is very little bloodflow in and around the tissue, so healing takes a long time. Trust me; you want to treat this injury right away.

SYMPTOMS

- Pain on the outside of the ankle just below the ankle bone that is worse during running and eases up when you stop
- Possible swelling, which may indicate a tear

WHAT'S GOING ON

There are two tendons that run along the outside of your ankle just behind the ankle bone and connect to the metatarsals of the foot. They are the peroneus longus and peroneus brevis tendons. When they repeatedly rub against the bone at your ankle, they become inflamed, and it hurts.

A big bump up in mileage can stress these tendons, especially if you underpronate or spend too much time on the outside of your rearfoot when you run. Picture this: As your foot lands on the ground,

PERONEUS BREVIS

PERONEUS LONGUS

the bottom of your heel turns inward as your ankle pushes outward against the peroneal tendons. When this gets repeated over and over again as you run, those tendons get irritated.

Tight peroneal muscles can play a role since they will pull the tendons tighter across the bone. And if you run frequently across sloped surfaces, your ankle is forced to extend outward and against the peroneal tendons, creating friction and leading to inflammation.

WHAT TO DO

(Instructions for the stretches and calf roll below appear at the end of this chapter.)

- Use dynamic rest to maintain your fitness until you can run comfortably without any changes to your running form. Swimming is great, but any cardio that doesn't hurt your ankle will do.

- Ice the sore area for 15 minutes four to six times a day.

- If you can stretch without pain, do straight-leg and bent-leg calf stretches daily.

- Use your foam roller to loosen your calf muscles.

- If discomfort lasts more than 10 days, see a sports doctor, who may recommend a walking boot or ankle brace. If a tear is suspected, she will order an MRI to see what's going on. In cases that don't improve with dynamic rest and conservative treatment, your doctor may recommend platelet-rich plasma injections.

PREVENTION

(Instructions for the stretches and exercises below appear at the end of this chapter.)

- Strengthen your peroneal muscles and calves by doing the foot eversion exercise and calf raises.

- Use your foam roller daily to keep muscles loose. Roll your calves, and then to hit the peroneals, turn your leg to roll the outside of it.

- To find out if you underpronate or supinate when you run, have a physical therapist, coach, or a staff person at your local running shop watch you run. If you underpronate, choose running shoes designed to help correct your foot motion and consider over-the-counter shoe inserts. I like heat-moldable ones, which you can find online. I link to the products I like through my Web site, drjordanmetzl.com. If those don't help, consider custom-made orthotics.

Ankle Sprain

You're running blissfully along a shaded trail or through an open meadow and suddenly—whoa!—your foot lands in a shallow hole and your ankle rolls.

SYMPTOMS

- Pain and swelling
- Possible bruising

  Sprains are graded according to the severity of symptoms.

- Grade 1: Tolerable pain, some swelling, and some difficulty walking
- Grade 2: Moderate pain, swelling, poor range of motion in your ankle
- Grade 3: Significant pain and swelling, bruising, and total joint instability (you will not be able to walk)

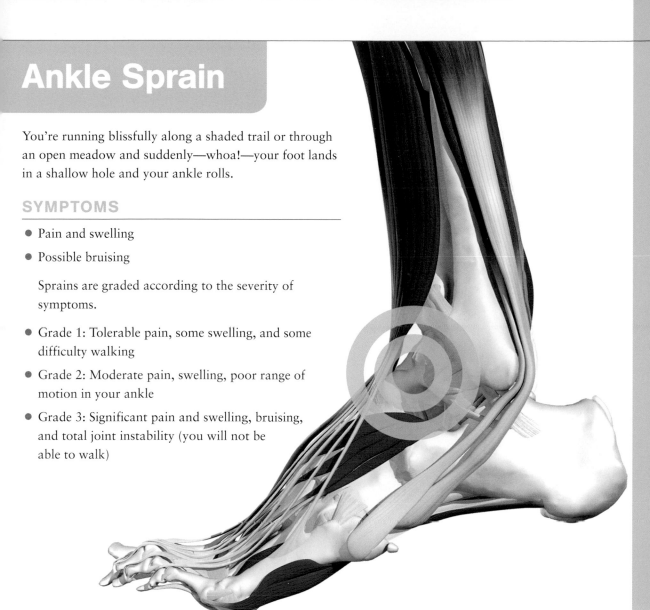

WHAT'S GOING ON

An ankle sprain is an injury to the ligaments around your ankle. In most cases a sprain results from rolling your ankle excessively outward. Less common is a medial sprain, which occurs when your foot rolls inward, injuring the ligaments on the inside of the ankle.

51

WHAT TO DO

- Stay fit with dynamic rest. Swimming or running in the pool are great, and keep doing your upper-body work.

- Ice and elevate your ankle to reduce swelling, but don't ice it for more than 15 minutes at a time.

- Take an anti-inflammatory, such as ibuprofen or naproxen, to reduce pain and inflammation.

- If pain and swelling are significant (grade 2 or 3 sprain), see a doctor. There may be damage to the tendons, cartilage, or bones of your foot, and a severe case may involve full tears of the ligaments as well as dislocation of the ankle.

- Crutches are a good idea for grade 2 or 3 sprains. As the sprain heals, compression with an elastic bandage can help with internal bleeding and swelling.

- When the pain becomes tolerable, perform some basic range-of-motion moves. During the first week do only the following: Pull your foot back toward your shin and then point it away in the opposite direction. Don't rotate your ankle or create any side-to-side movement, which will aggravate injured ligaments. After the first week, you can add in rotation: Do ankle rotations in one direction and then the other. Go slowly to start, especially if your ankle is still sore, and increase the speed and reps as your injury heals. This exercise will help your ankle return to full range of motion.

- With an ankle injury, your calf muscles tighten to prevent your ankle from moving, so do some simple stretches to keep your calves loose. You don't want to strain them when you return to running.

PREVENTION

You can't totally prevent an ankle sprain, but you can increase ankle stability and improve your balance to keep from rolling or twisting an ankle. (Instructions for the stretches and exercises below appear at the end of this chapter.)

- Build strength and stability by doing the IronStrength workout (see Chapter 12 for the exercises and videos) once or twice a week and plyometric jump squats, lunges, and zigzags daily.

- Maintain flexibility in your calves with the calf roll, straight-leg calf stretch, and bent-leg calf stretch.

- Improve ankle stability by regularly balancing on one foot. Challenge yourself by moving your arms, twisting your upper body, or bending at the knee. Want to take it to the next level? Try balancing on one foot while your eyes are closed. Be sure to work both sides equally to prevent an imbalance.

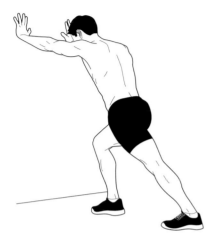

STRETCHES

STRAIGHT-LEG CALF STRETCHES

Stand facing a wall with your arms straight in front of you and your hands flat against the wall. Keep your right leg forward, foot flat on the floor, and extend your left leg straight back, placing your heel flat on the floor. Don't bend your back knee. Lean into the wall until you feel the stretch in the calf of the straight leg. Hold for 30 seconds and switch sides. Repeat twice for a total of 3 sets. Perform this stretch daily and up to three times a day if you are really tight.

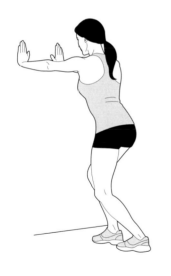

BENT-LEG CALF STRETCHES

Stand facing a wall with your arms straight in front of you and your hands flat against the wall. Keep your right leg forward, foot flat on the floor. Move your left leg back until the toes of your left foot are even with the heel of your front foot. Make sure the heels of both feet are down against the floor. Now bend at your knees until you feel a comfortable stretch just above your ankle. Hold for 30 seconds and switch sides. Repeat twice for a total of three sets. Perform this stretch daily and up to three times a day if you are really tight.

FOAM ROLLER EXERCISES

CALF ROLLS

Seated on the floor, place a foam roller under your right ankle. Cross your left leg over your right. Place your hands flat on the floor for support and keep your back naturally arched. Roll your body forward until the roller reaches the back of your right knee; then roll back and forth from knee to ankle 15 times. Repeat with the left leg. Do 3 sets daily. If this is too difficult, you can perform the movement with both legs on the roller.

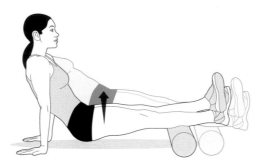

STRENGTH EXERCISES

FOOT EVERSIONS WITH A RESISTANCE BAND

Anchor one end of a resistance band to a sturdy structure, like the leg of a sofa. Sit on the floor and place the other end of the band around your foot so it is taut against the outside of that foot; then straighten your leg and without moving it push your foot outward against the band. Repeat 10 to 20 times and switch sides. Do 3 sets daily.

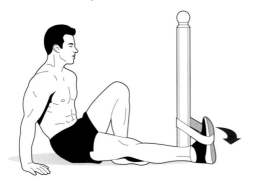

ECCENTRIC CALF RAISES

Stand on a step with your heels hanging off the edge. Holding on to the rail, first push yourself up (concentric movement), then very slowly—to the count of 10 seconds—drop your heels below the level of your feet (eccentric strengthening). Push back up and repeat. Do 3 sets of 15 every day.

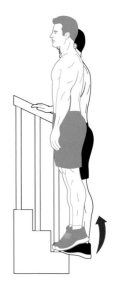

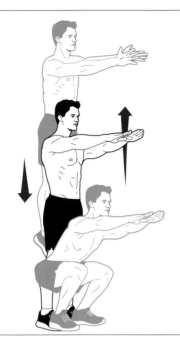

PLYOMETRIC JUMP SQUATS

Stand tall with your feet a little more than shoulder-width apart and toes turned slightly outward. Put your arms straight out in front of you. Squat down, pushing your butt back while keeping your upper body tall. (If you can get your butt down below your knees, you will give your glutes an extra-good workout.) Now explode up as high as you can and land softly. Maintain good anatomical position and keep the motion controlled, landing softly on your heels after each jump. Do 3 sets of 15 daily.

STEP INSIDE THE GYM WITH ME

To watch a video showing how to do plyometric jump squats, turn to page 200.

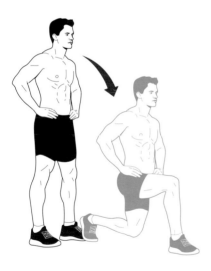

LUNGES

Stand tall, keeping your trunk upright and stable, and lunge forward with your right leg as you lower your body until your back knee nearly touches the ground. Pause, and then push yourself back to the starting position. Engage your core muscles to keep your upper body stable and upright; you don't want to bend forward or side to side. Complete 10 reps and switch sides, lunging with your left leg. Do 3 sets daily (1 set equals a right and left lunge).

ZIGZAGS

To improve ankle mobility and stability, change directions when you run. Run figure-8 drills, use cones to create obstacle runs or draw obstacles on a driveway with chalk, add direction changes to your interval workouts, or find an empty parking lot and run patterns in and out and around the parking spaces.

CHAPTER 5

YOUR LOWER LEGS

Next up the kinetic chain are your lower legs—home of your calves, shins, and Achilles tendons, named for the Greek god Achilles, whose weakness was his heel.

And though the Achilles can be *your* weakness if injured, it is what makes you a distance runner. This tendon, which connects your calf muscles to your heel, works like a spring, storing and releasing energy as you run. Our primate relatives—chimpanzees, monkeys, gorillas—do not have an Achilles tendon; their calves connect directly to their heels, making them lousy runners on two legs. Who would win a two-legged race, you or a chimp? You would. So be kind to your Achilles and its kinetic chain partner, your calf.

Where Does It Hurt?

1. Pain anywhere along the Achilles tendon, from your heel to your calf, indicates *Achilles tendonitis.*

2. If you feel soreness or achiness along your shin during running, you have *shin splints*, an umbrella term that covers *stress injuries* to the bone, *stress fractures* of the bone, and *compartment syndrome*, a muscular malady.

3. Pain in your calf signals a *calf strain.* During your run, you may experience anything from a twinge followed by discomfort and tightness on up to a blast of sharp excruciating pain after which your muscle will not work.

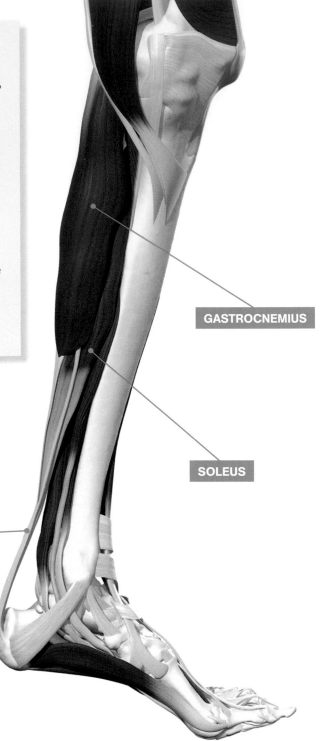

GASTROCNEMIUS

SOLEUS

ACHILLES TENDON

Achilles Tendonitis

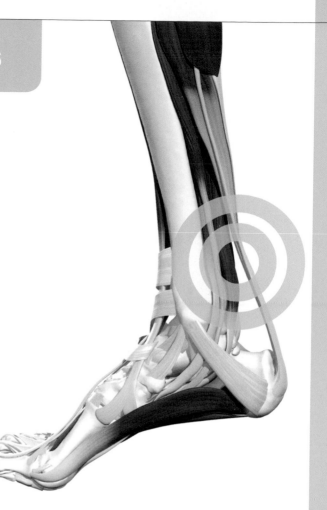

The Achilles tendon is one tough piece of tissue, but not so tough that it can't get hurt—and once it gets sore, it stays sore for a very long time. If you ignore this injury, it will turn into tendonosis, and if that sounds nasty, it is: You very well might end up with a torn Achilles and a long, long layoff from running.

SYMPTOMS

- Mild to severe soreness anywhere from the back of your heel up to where your tendon meets your calf muscles at the muscle–tendon junction, which forms a V at the base of your calf
- A lump in the tendon, which is a sign of a tear

WHAT'S GOING ON

Achilles tendonitis is a classic overuse injury. It results from ramping up your mileage, intensity, or hill running too quickly, but there are other factors that come into play.

- Having weak calf muscles makes your Achilles tendon vulnerable because it will be forced to take on more of the load of running.
- Tight calf muscles create greater tension along your Achilles, upping your risk of injury.
- If you overpronate, your Achilles will be pulled out of ideal alignment, which puts extra stress on the tendon.

STEP INTO MY OFFICE
Blipp this page to view
a video about
Achilles tendonitis.

- If you overstride, you land on the ground farther from the center of your body mass, which increases the forces traveling up your legs.

Too much stress on a tendon overburdened by weak calves or poor running mechanics breaks down the collagen fibers that make up the tendon and messes up their alignment. Chronic irritation leads to fluid buildup in the tendon, called tendonosis, and the tissue may eventually tear.

Take care of Achilles soreness right away and you will be running painfree again in 6 to 10 weeks. Ignore it and you are looking at 3 to 6 months of recovery, maybe even longer. Why so long? There is very little bloodflow in and around tendons, and bloodflow speeds healing.

WHAT TO DO

(Instructions for the stretches and exercises below appear at the end of this chapter.)

- Use dynamic rest: Swim, bike, run in the pool. Do anything that you can do pain-free, but do not run. And be sure to keep up with upper-body strength training.

- Ice the sore area for 15 minutes four to six times a day.

- If you can stretch without pain, do straight-leg and bent-leg calf stretches.

- Use your foam roller to loosen your calf muscles, making sure not to go below the calf onto your sore tendon.

- Perform some eccentric strengthening by doing eccentric calf raises. An eccentric exercise is one in which your muscle lengthens while you are loading it. With an Achilles injury, this not only strengthens the calf muscle and tendon but also helps to heal the tendon by stimulating collagen production and realigning the collagen fibers.

- Make sure you are getting all the nutrients you need. Vitamin C, manganese, and zinc play an important role in making collagen, and vitamins B_6 and E have been linked to tendon health. A well-balanced diet rich in fruits and vegetables, whole grains, and lean protein will supply sufficient amounts of these vitamins; if your diet is not of the healthy kind, consider seeing a nutritionist.

- See your doctor if you have a lump in your tendon, if your pain lasts for more than several days, or if discomfort has caused you to limp or alter your running form.

PREVENTION

The key to preventing Achilles tendonitis, as with all injuries, really, is to figure out the underlying cause and focus on correcting it.

- Strengthen your calves so they can take on more of the load of running rather than force your tendons to take on too much. Stay faithful to the IronStrength workout (see Chapter 12 and watch the videos) once or twice a week, and do plyometric lunges, single-leg standing dumbbell calf raises, single-leg bent-knee calf raises, and the farmer's walk on toes (all shown at the end of this chapter) every day.

- Also add in plenty of plyometric lower-body work, like squats, multidirectional lunges, squat thrusts, and so on.

- Keep your calves from becoming too tight by using your foam roller daily.

- Check your stride. While running, count how many times your right foot strikes the ground in 60 seconds. You want to hit between 85 and 90 times. Lower than that indicates a longer stride, which increases the load on your legs. A shorter, quicker stride can help prevent injury.

- Check your foot motion: Have a coach, physical therapist, or even a staff person at your local running shop watch you run to see if you overpronate. If you do, choose shoes that offer good medial support or try over-the-counter orthotics. I like heat-moldable inserts, which you can find online.

- Remember to follow the 10 percent rule: Don't increase your mileage by more than 10 percent each week.

Shin Splints

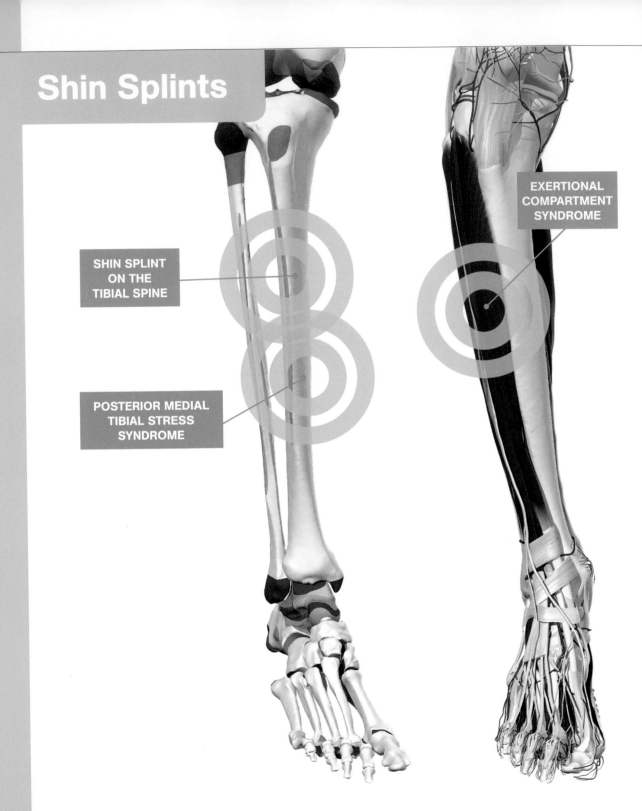

SHIN SPLINT
ON THE
TIBIAL SPINE

POSTERIOR MEDIAL
TIBIAL STRESS
SYNDROME

EXERTIONAL
COMPARTMENT
SYNDROME

Shin splints are so common that either you or almost any runner you know has had them at some point. But this phrase gets thrown around so loosely that nobody really knows what shin splints actually are. The truth is there are different types of shin pain, all of which are called shin splints. These include muscular and bone-related shin pain. Let's have a look at how we can make more sense out of your achy shins.

SYMPTOMS

Roughly 90 percent of shin splints occur in the bone.

If you feel an achy pain *along the inside* of your shinbone (the tibia) when you run, you likely have posterior medial tibial stress syndrome. After running, push on your bone in the tender area; if pressing on the bone hurts, you indeed have a stressed-out tibia.

If you feel pain *along the front* of your shinbone, on the sharp part of the tibia called the tibial spine, during running and when you press on the bone, see your doctor right away. I rarely see this, but it is more serious. Here's why: Your tibia is built like a bow; it flexes as you put pressure on it. The front of your tibia is the tension side of the bow, and a shin splint there can widen and quickly turn into a stress fracture.

How do you know if you have a stress fracture? Only your doctor can tell for sure, but if as you're pressing your fingers into your shinbone you can locate a specific point that elicits a sharp pain, you probably have a stress fracture. See your doc.

If you feel a *tightening pain* in the softer muscular tissue toward the outside of your tibia, you probably have exertional compartment syndrome (ECS). This pain only occurs while you're running and isn't present when you are at rest. Runners who get this tell me it feels like their muscles want to pop out of their skin when they run. ECS makes up about 10 percent of shin splints, and though it almost always happens in the front of your lower leg, it can also occur in the back.

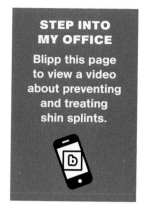

STEP INTO MY OFFICE

Blipp this page to view a video about preventing and treating shin splints.

WHAT'S GOING ON

Bone-Related

Bone-related shin splints occur when there is simply more load or stress on the tibia than it can handle. They are common among new runners who are just beginning to adapt to the demands of the sport. In response to the stress of running, bone becomes stronger, but it takes time. Experienced runners get shin splints when they ramp up their running too quickly. When you increase the workload significantly and your bone isn't ready for the extra load, it literally becomes irritated. When your tibia calls out in pain, pay attention. Initially what you have is a *stress response* or *stress injury,* but if you continue to run and the bone becomes increasingly irritated, it swells and eventually cracks—and then you've got a *stress fracture.*

In addition to overeager training, poor body mechanics (your foot type, footstrike, hip motion), wearing running shoes that aren't right for you, and low bone density can contribute to the development of bone-related shin splints.

Muscle-Related

ECS results from swelling within a compartment in your lower leg. A compartment consists of a muscle, nerves, and blood vessels wrapped in a tough membrane called *fascia.* Your lower leg has four of them. The anterior compartment is at the front of your leg. Because fascia's job is to hold your muscles in place, it's not very flexible, and when the tissue within the compartment swells, it pushes against the fascia, causing pain. As with bone-related shin splints, a sudden increase in running, wearing the wrong shoes, and poor body mechanics can lead to a buildup of stress that, in this case, causes swelling in your muscle.

DO YOU HAVE WEAK BONES?

Because if you do, you are at greater risk than the average runner for stress fractures. Here's a checklist of the characteristics of someone who is more likely to have low bone density.

- Female
- Of northern European descent: blond hair, blue eyes, pale skin
- Thin body type
- Female who has experienced amenorrhea (missed three or more menstrual cycles in a row)
- Diet low in calcium and vitamin D

WHAT TO DO

If the pain is mild and you can run without altering your running mechanics, keep going. If you are changing the way you run to accommodate the pain, you need to take a break from running and get healthy. But stay active and fit with swimming, cycling, the elliptical—any non-weight-bearing activity—and continue with upper-body strength training.

Bone-Related

- Apply ice to the area for 15 minutes four to six times a day.

- If the pain forces you to change the way you run, stop running and see a sports doctor for a proper diagnosis. Stress injuries can become stress fractures, which can sideline you for a long time. Your doctor will order an x-ray or MRI. Typically stress fractures don't show up on x-rays unless they are well on their way to cracking (very serious) or already in the healing stage, during which the body makes a callus—a bump on the bone at the site of the injury.

- If your doctor assures you that you do not have a stress fracture, you can take an anti-inflammatory, such as ibuprofen or naproxen, but don't take one if you don't have a diagnosis. Anti-inflammatories mask the pain, and if you keep running on a stressed tibia, you could end up with a stress fracture.

- If the tests come back confirming a stress fracture, your doctor may also request a bone density scan depending on your case and family history.

- Talk with your doctor to try to figure out what caused your injury so you can begin to put into place strategies that will help you heal and prevent a recurrence.

- If you overpronate, try over-the-counter arch supports. I like heat-moldable inserts; you can find lots of options online. If they don't work and you continue to get stress fractures, consider custom orthotics.

- If your diet is low in calcium, eat more calcium- and vitamin D–rich foods. Dairy products are the best sources (see Chapter 15 for other options).

Muscle-Related

- Use a foam roller on your shins and calves, as shown at the end of this chapter, for several minutes at a time several times a day to loosen the fascia. Manual massage can help as well.

- Wear motion-control shoes or try arch supports to help correct biomechanical problems in your feet and take stress off the affected muscles.

- If these measures don't help, see a sports doctor, who may do a test using a needle to measure the pressure inside your leg before and after you run. If the difference in pressure is high, a surgical procedure called a fasciotomy can be performed to open the fascia and allow it to expand. This procedure is rarely performed, however.

PREVENTION

Bone-Related

- Follow the 10 percent rule—increase mileage no more than 10 percent from week to week. If you are brand new to running, start with a walk/run combination for 30 minutes several times a week, increasing the run portion and shortening the walk until you can run comfortably for 30 minutes.

- Overpronation loads more force onto the inner side of the tibia. If you overpronate, wear a running shoe with a medial post or try arch supports.

- Strengthen your kinetic chain by doing the IronStrength workout once or twice a week (see Chapter 12 and watch the videos). Good strength in your hips and core improves your running alignment and reduces the load on your shins.

- Shorten your stride and increase your cadence. This changes the mechanics of your running to put less load on your feet, shins, and everything up your kinetic chain. Count every time your feet strike the ground for 1 minute. Aim for 170 to 180 footstrikes.

- Make sure you get enough calcium and vitamin D daily: 1,000 milligrams of calcium (women over 50 and men over 70 need 1,200 milligrams); 600 IU of vitamin D (all adults over 70 need 800 IU). The best sources are dairy products (see Chapter 15 for other options).

Muscle-Related

- Use the foam roller on your shins and calves daily as shown at the end of this chapter, and consider getting a massage once or twice a month.

- Wear motion-control running shoes or try arch supports.

CASE STUDY: LAUREN FONTANA

Stats: Lauren is a college student who runs cross-country and track.

Complaint: She came to me to find out what was going on with her shins. She had a history of shin splints since high school, but this was different. When she was walking, everything felt fine, but during running, she developed pain in her shins that became so severe her legs would tighten up and she would be forced to stop. Sometimes she even found it difficult to stand.

Diagnosis: The tightness that Lauren described and the fact that it didn't hurt to walk suggested to me that she probably had exertional compartment syndrome, so I did pressure testing, which confirmed the diagnosis.

Treatment: Because Lauren's case was so severe, I recommended she get surgery—a fasciotomy—which she did. Afterward I ordered 2 weeks of complete rest, and then I gave her the green light to gradually return to running, along with daily foam-rolling before and after every run and regular IronStrength workouts.

Outcome: Lauren and I are both thrilled to report that she achieved 100 percent recovery and is running strong and pain-free.

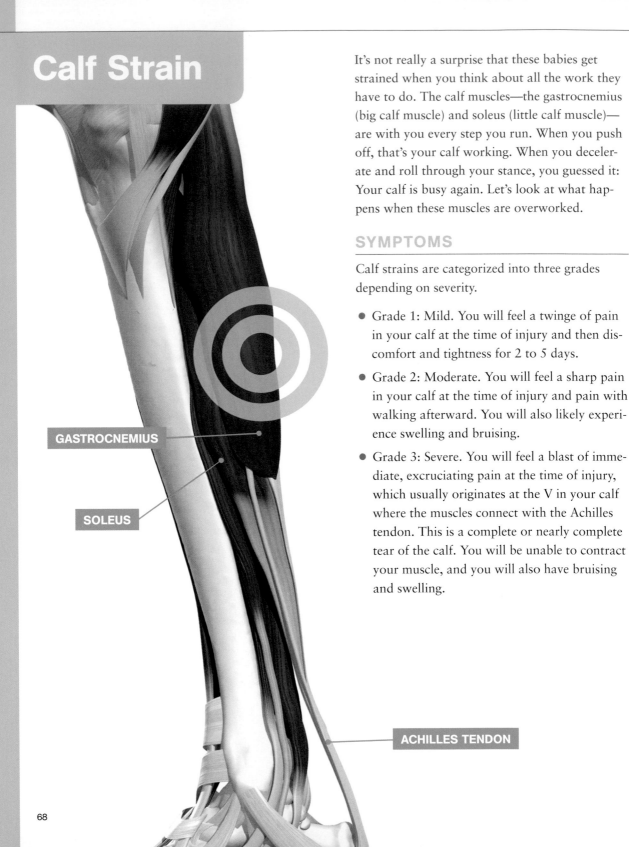

Calf Strain

It's not really a surprise that these babies get strained when you think about all the work they have to do. The calf muscles—the gastrocnemius (big calf muscle) and soleus (little calf muscle)—are with you every step you run. When you push off, that's your calf working. When you decelerate and roll through your stance, you guessed it: Your calf is busy again. Let's look at what happens when these muscles are overworked.

SYMPTOMS

Calf strains are categorized into three grades depending on severity.

- Grade 1: Mild. You will feel a twinge of pain in your calf at the time of injury and then discomfort and tightness for 2 to 5 days.

- Grade 2: Moderate. You will feel a sharp pain in your calf at the time of injury and pain with walking afterward. You will also likely experience swelling and bruising.

- Grade 3: Severe. You will feel a blast of immediate, excruciating pain at the time of injury, which usually originates at the V in your calf where the muscles connect with the Achilles tendon. This is a complete or nearly complete tear of the calf. You will be unable to contract your muscle, and you will also have bruising and swelling.

GASTROCNEMIUS

SOLEUS

ACHILLES TENDON

WHAT'S GOING ON

Calf strains occur when you push off fast from the ground and your muscle isn't ready for the explosive effort. Maybe you have dashed into a speed workout or blasted off the starting line of a 5-K without warming up first.

Weak or tight calves are particularly vulnerable to strains. In a mild (grade 1) strain, up to 10 percent of muscle fibers are torn. With a grade 2 strain, up to 90 percent of muscle is torn. Grade 3? Bad news.

WHAT TO DO

Treat a calf strain as soon as possible after it occurs. If you neglect it or continue to run through it, you will make it worse and then suffer a longer layoff.

- Sorry, no running. For that matter, all activities involving the lower leg are off-limits. But you can continue with upper-body strength training.

- Ice your muscles for 15 to 20 minutes four to six times during the first 24 hours. This will help reduce pain, inflammation, and muscle spasms.

- Compression for the first 24 to 48 hours after injury can help keep swelling down. The easiest way is to use a compression sleeve. You can also wrap your calf with elastic bandages, but be careful not to wrap it too tightly; if your foot turns color or gets cold, bloodflow has been overly restricted and you need to loosen the bandage.

- Elevate your lower leg above you hip as much as possible during the first 48 hours after injuring your calf. This will help draw fluid away from the injury and prevent excessive swelling.

- For the first couple days after the injury, use heel pads in your shoes to raise your heel, shortening your calf and reducing strain on the muscles.

- An anti-inflammatory, such as ibuprofen or naproxen, may help reduce pain and inflammation.

- If you have a grade 2 or 3 strain, or if your symptoms don't improve, see your doctor. She will be able to determine the severity of your injury and diagnose any underlying problems. She may also prescribe physical therapy. If you have ruptured your calf lower down near your Achilles tendon, surgery may be recommended and usually results in a full recovery. But know that calf injuries are almost always treated nonsurgically.

REHABILITATION

Once you can walk without pain, it is important to rehabilitate your calf muscles before you return to running, or you risk straining your calf again. Rehabilitation involves stretching to help lengthen the scar tissue that forms during healing and strengthening to get your calf in shape for running.

Stretch

- To stretch the gastrocnemius (big muscle), sit on the floor with your leg straight out in front of you. Pull your toes and foot back toward you and hold for several seconds. Relax and repeat for a total of 10 reps, and then switch legs.

- To stretch the soleus (smaller muscle), sit on the floor with your knees bent. Place your hands on the floor behind you, supporting yourself on your arms as you lean back. Lift your leg, keeping it bent, and point your toes toward the ceiling. Hold for several seconds. Relax and repeat for a total of 10 reps, and then switch legs.

Strengthen

- Sit on the floor with your leg straight out in front of you. Use a resistance band or a towel placed across the ball of your foot for resistance, and point your foot away from your body. Pause; relax and repeat. Do 3 sets of 15.

- Do single-leg calf raises: Stand on a step with your heels hanging off the edge. Holding on to the rail, first push yourself up on one leg, and then very slowly—to the count of 10 seconds—drop your heels below the level of your feet. Push back up and repeat. Do 3 sets of 15.

PREVENTION

(Instructions for the stretches and exercises below appear at the end of this chapter.)

- Keep your calf muscles loose. Think about it: It's much harder to rip something pliable, like a rubber band. (I'm not saying you want rubber band muscles, because you don't—more on that later—but you do want a little flexibility.) Use your foam roller daily, and also perform the calf roll, straight-leg calf stretch, and bent-leg calf stretch a few times a day.

- Strengthen your entire kinetic chain by doing the IronStrength workout (see Chapter 12 and watch the videos) once or twice a week and do the single-leg standing dumbbell calf raises, single-leg bent-knee calf raises, and the farmer's walk on toes daily.

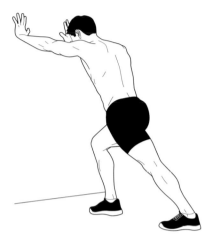

STRETCHES

STRAIGHT-LEG CALF STRETCHES

Stand facing a wall with your arms straight in front of you and your hands flat against the wall. Keep your right leg forward, foot flat on the floor, and extend your left leg straight back, placing your heel flat on the floor. Don't bend your back knee. Lean into the wall until you feel the stretch in the calf of the straight leg. Hold for 30 seconds and switch sides. Repeat twice for a total of 3 sets. Perform this stretch daily and up to three times a day if you are really tight.

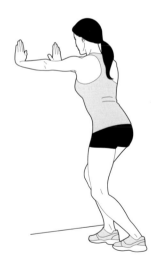

BENT-LEG CALF STRETCHES

Stand facing a wall with your arms straight in front of you and your hands flat against the wall. Keep your right leg forward, foot flat on the floor. Move your left leg back until the toes of your left foot are even with the heel of your front foot. Make sure the heels of both feet are down against the floor. Now bend at your knees until you feel a comfortable stretch just above your ankle. Hold for 30 seconds and switch sides. Repeat twice for a total of 3 sets. Perform this stretch daily and up to three times a day if you are really tight.

FOAM ROLLER EXERCISES

SHIN ROLLS

Facing the floor, place a foam roller at the top of your shins below your knees. Supporting your body with your hands on the floor beneath your shoulders, roll your shin back and forth over the roller from knee to ankle several times. Repeat with your other leg.

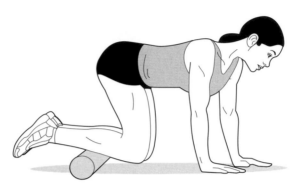

CALF ROLLS

Seated on the floor with your right leg straight in front of you, place a foam roller under your right ankle. Cross your left leg over your right ankle. Place your hands flat on the floor for support and keep your back naturally arched. Roll your body forward until the roller reaches the back of your right knee; then roll back and forth from knee to ankle several times. Repeat with the left leg. If this is too difficult, you can perform the movement with both legs on the roller.

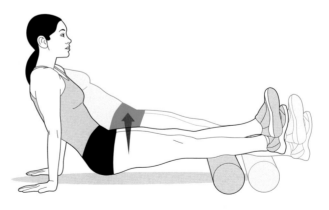

STRENGTH EXERCISES

STEP INSIDE THE GYM WITH ME

To watch a video showing how to do plyometric lunges, turn to page 203.

ECCENTRIC CALF RAISES

Stand on a step with your heels hanging off the edge. Holding on to the rail, first push yourself up (concentric movement), and then very slowly—to the count of 10 seconds—drop your heels below the level of your feet (eccentric strengthening). Push back up and repeat. Do 3 sets of 15 daily.

PLYOMETRIC LUNGES

Stand with your feet together, and then lunge forward with your right foot and left arm until the shin of your back leg is parallel to the floor and your knee almost touches. Push back to the starting position. Do the same with your opposite leg and arm. Now do the same movement, but switch your legs in midair: Lunge forward with your right foot and push explosively off the floor, switching legs in midair to lunge forward with your left. Left and right count as 1 rep. It is important to control your motion as you do this exercise; keep your trunk upright and your pelvis stable. You shouldn't be flailing around. Do 3 sets of 15 reps daily and up to 5 sets of 15 if you're advanced. If this move is too difficult, start with isometric lunges—taking out the jump—and as you become proficient at those, graduate to plyometric lunges.

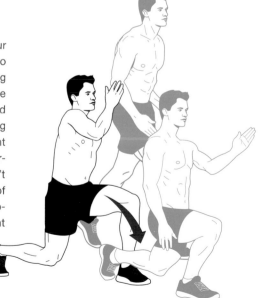

73

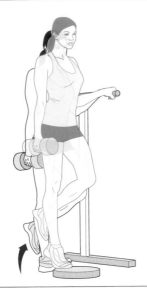

SINGLE-LEG STANDING DUMBBELL CALF RAISES

Holding a dumbbell in your right hand, stand on a step or block. Cross your left foot behind your right ankle, balance on the ball of your right foot, and let your heel hang over the edge of the step. Put your left hand on a rail or against the wall for stability. Lift your right heel as high as you can and pause; then lower and repeat. Complete 15 reps and then switch sides, holding the dumbbell in your left hand. Do 3 sets of 15 reps on each side daily.

SINGLE-LEG BENT-KNEE CALF RAISES

Follow the instructions for the single-leg standing dumbbell calf raises, but bend the knee of your balancing leg and keep it bent as you raise and lower your body. Do 15 reps and switch sides. Complete 3 sets of 15 reps on each side daily.

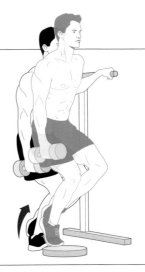

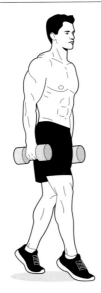

FARMER'S WALK ON TOES

Hold a pair of heavy dumbbells straight down at your sides. Rise up on your toes and walk forward for 60 seconds. Be sure to stand tall as you perform this exercise. This move not only works your calves but also improves your cardiovascular fitness. Choose the heaviest pair of dumbbells that allows you to perform this exercise without breaking form for 60 seconds. If you feel that you could have gone longer, grab heavier weights on your next set. Do 3 sets daily.

CHAPTER 6

YOUR KNEES

If you come spend a day in my office, you will see plenty of runners lining the halls with their achy knees.

Many are freaked out before they get to my office: Is my running career over? Can I still run? Is it time to start swimming for the rest of my life?

Thankfully, the vast majority of knee injuries are not going to keep you off the road for an extended period of time. In this section, I'm going to tell you how to recognize and prevent the most common types of knee problems that befall runners.

Runner's Knee
(aka Patellofemoral Knee Pain)

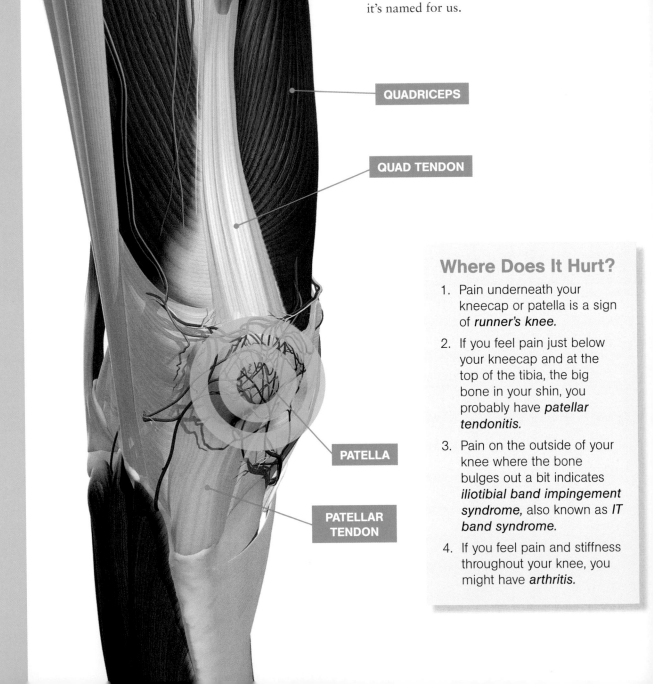

This injury is so common among runners that it's named for us.

QUADRICEPS

QUAD TENDON

PATELLA

PATELLAR TENDON

Where Does It Hurt?

1. Pain underneath your kneecap or patella is a sign of *runner's knee.*

2. If you feel pain just below your kneecap and at the top of the tibia, the big bone in your shin, you probably have *patellar tendonitis.*

3. Pain on the outside of your knee where the bone bulges out a bit indicates *iliotibial band impingement syndrome,* also known as *IT band syndrome.*

4. If you feel pain and stiffness throughout your knee, you might have *arthritis.*

SYMPTOMS

- An achy pain underneath your kneecap that is worse after running but may flare up after about an hour of running when your quadriceps (muscles of the front of the thigh) start to tire
- Especially painful when you go up or down stairs

STEP INTO MY OFFICE

Blipp this page to view a video about prevention and treatment of runner's knee.

WHAT'S GOING ON

The patella sits between two tendons: the quadriceps tendon above, which connects to the quadriceps muscle, and the patellar tendon below, which attaches to the tibia. The underside of the patella is covered in articular cartilage, which allows smooth movement of the kneecap over the joint in a groove called the trochlea. (Articular cartilage is not to be confused with the meniscus cartilage that cushions the area between tibia and femur.) When the patella moves out of alignment over and over again during running, the articular cartilage beneath the patella becomes irritated.

There are several ways that the patella can be derailed.

- Since the patella is literally connected to the quadriceps, tightness or weakness in those muscles affects the movement of the kneecap.
- Your foot mechanics may be the cause: Overpronation increases stress along the inside of the patella.
- If your hip and core muscles are weak, your hip will drop as you run, which then causes your knee to collapse inward.

WHAT TO DO

I generally let people with runner's knee stay on the road unless they're limping like an old dog. The key here is to try to reduce the pain while simultaneously figuring out why the injury happened.

- Ice your knee for 15 minutes four to six times a day.
- Take an anti-inflammatory, such as naproxen or ibuprofen, to ease the pain.
- Use your foam roller to loosen tight quads and a tight IT band as shown at the end of this chapter.

- If you are still in pain after 2 months of rest and TLC, or if swelling develops, you may have a different problem; see your doctor. He may recommend an MRI to look at the cartilage.
- Older than 50? See your doctor to rule out patellofemoral arthritis—a wearing down of the cartilage beneath the kneecap.

PREVENTION

The best way to prevent runner's knee is with a strong and healthy kinetic chain. (Instructions for the exercises below appear at the end of this chapter.)

- Strengthen the muscles in your quads, hips, glutes, and core. Strong quadriceps will help stabilize your knee, and strong hips, glutes, and core muscles provide stability, preventing your hip from dropping and your knee from caving inward as you run. I love plyometric jump squats along with mountain climbers and walking lunges. And don't forget to do the IronStrength workout once or twice a week (see Chapter 12 and watch the videos).

- Use your foam roller daily to keep muscles loose, and add 2 extra sets of the quad roll and the ITB roll.

- Have a coach, physical therapist, or staff member from your local running store watch you run to check pronation. If you overpronate, wear running shoes that have medial support to correct the motion; if shoes alone don't help, try over-the-counter orthotics. My preference is heat-moldable inserts, which you can order online.

- A shorter, quicker stride reduces the loading force to your leg. Count every time your feet hit the ground for a minute and aim for 170 to 180 footstrikes.

Patellar Tendonitis

Common in athletes who play basketball and other sports that require lots of jumping, this injury also goes by the name jumper's knee. But runners guilty of doing too much too soon, especially cruising lots of downhills, can fall victim to this malady as well.

SYMPTOMS

- Pain just below the kneecap and at the top of the tibia (shinbone) that sharpens during running

- As it progresses, pain when going up and down stairs

WHAT'S GOING ON

A tendon is the ropelike structure that connects muscle to bone. In the case of the knee, the patellar tendon connects the strong muscles of the quadriceps to the tibia. Due to the large loading forces across the knee associated with running, patellar loading forces can sometimes be too much for the tendon and can cause irritation, called tendonitis. Left untreated, chronic tendonitis can turn into a more stubborn problem called tendonosis. And persistent tendonosis can lead to a degenerative partial tear of the tendon.

WHAT TO DO

- You need to lay off running until you can run free of pain, so use dynamic rest. Swim if you can without pain, and continue to do upper-body strengthening exercises.

- Apply ice for 15 minutes four to six times a day to help relieve pain.

- Try massaging the area to ease pain and promote healing.

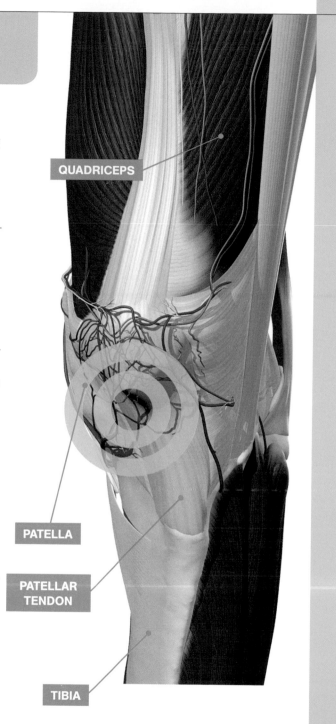

QUADRICEPS

PATELLA

PATELLAR TENDON

TIBIA

- Consider a patellar tendon strap, which wraps around your leg just under the knee to support the tendon and help reduce pain.

- If you don't notice improvement in 3 weeks, see your doctor, who may prescribe anti-inflammatories and physical therapy. For severe cases, your doc may recommend an injection of platelet-rich plasma (see "PRP: Cutting-Edge Treatment" on page 36 to learn more).

- Rehabilitate your leg before you return to running using the strength exercises recommended for prevention, below.

PREVENTION

(Instructions for the leg extension and the quad roll appear at the end of this chapter.)

- I am generally not a fan of the leg extension machine because it doesn't mimic real-life movement, but it can be effective in preventing a recurrence of patellar tendonitis. Slow lowering of the weight on the leg extension machine does a good job of strengthening the patellar tendon and the muscles around it.

- Stretch your quadriceps and hamstrings. When these muscles are tight, extra stress is loaded onto your tendon.

- Do the IronStrength workout once or twice a week to build total-body strength (see Chapter 12 and watch the videos).

- Use your foam roller daily to keep muscles loose (see page 210), and add 2 extra sets of the quad roll.

- Follow the 10 percent rule: Don't increase mileage more than 10 percent each week. This helps your body to adapt to the stresses of running and avoid injury.

Iliotibial Band Impingement Syndrome

If you came to my office, you would find more than a few runners every day with this exact story: "Dr. Metzl, I was running along and I was okay; then the outside of my knee started to hurt and pretty soon it felt like someone was jabbing a screwdriver into my knee."

It doesn't take long to recognize this injury, usually referred to by its acronym but also known as the dreaded iliotibial band (ITB) syndrome.

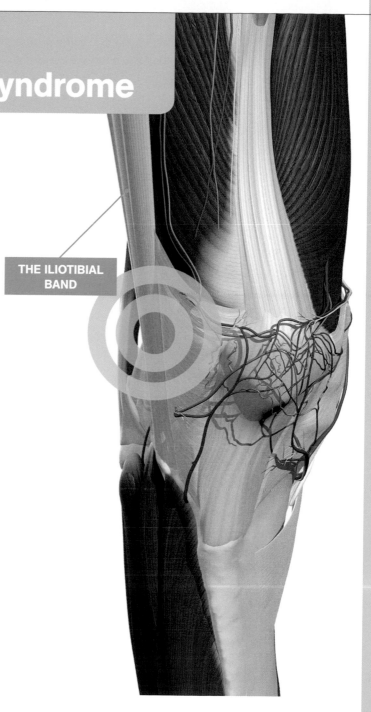

THE ILIOTIBIAL BAND

SYMPTOMS

- You will feel pain on the outer side of your knee where the bone bulges out that comes on anywhere from 5 to 7 minutes into your run and then subsides after you have stopped. You won't feel it while walking or during your day-to-day activities. It's easy to confuse ITB syndrome with a lateral meniscus tear, but here's how you tell the difference: Pain from the meniscus tear is located lower on the knee and is associated with a clicking sensation and swelling; the iliotibial band does not swell. Also, you will feel meniscus-tear pain during walking and other activities.

WHAT'S GOING ON

The iliotibial band is a tendon that connects the tensor fascia latae muscle, which originates on the outer side of your hip, to the tibia—the major bone in your lower leg. The ITB runs from your hip to your knee and crosses the knee joint. Its job is to help control the angle of your lower leg during running.

Now let's zoom in on your knee. A small, fluid-filled sac called the bursa sits between the ITB and the outside of your femur near your knee. When the ITB is tight, tension increases and the bursa gets squeezed. Over time the bursa swells and causes pain as you run.

There are several possible causes of ITB impingement syndrome.

- Weak muscles in your glutes and core allow your hips to drop when you run. I call this "doing the salsa." When that happens, your knee caves inward and tension increases along the ITB.

- Overpronation affects the movement around your knee, which stresses the ITB.

- Finally, ITB syndrome may result simply from a tight IT band.

WHAT TO DO

(Instructions for the exercises below appear at the end of this chapter.)

- You can run up to the point of pain or until pain forces a change in your form. Supplement your running with cycling, swimming, or another activity to maintain your cardiovascular fitness, and continue with strength training as comfort allows.

- Use your foam roller to loosen your ITB. Warning: Rolling your ITB is going to hurt—a lot—but this is normal. It means that the tendon is tight. Stay with it, rolling your ITB every day for 2 to 3 minutes on both legs.

- Strengthen your glutes and core to improve stability during running, which will help take stress off your ITB. Plyometric jump squats are terrific glute-strengtheners, and planks

work wonders on your core. Try to do 3 minutes of planks a day— 1 minute in the standard parallel-to-the-floor position and 1 minute on each side. And do 4 sets of 15 plyometric jump squats three or four times a week.

- If you overpronate, wear motion-control running shoes or try over-the-counter arch supports. I like heat-moldable orthotics, which you can find online.

- If you just can't seem to recover from this injury, see your doctor. She may prescribe physical therapy or recommend a cortisone shot into the bursa to reduce swelling. ITB syndrome responds well to cortisone, so don't be afraid to give it a try if nothing else is working.

PREVENTION

A strong butt and core are key to a happy running life and to preventing this injury. These muscles help stabilize your hips as you run. (Instructions for the exercises below appear at the end of this chapter.)

- Do the IronStrength workout once or twice a week (see Chapter 12 and watch the videos) as well as hip raises, reverse hip raises, low side-to-side lunges, the standing resistance-band hip abduction, and lateral band walks.

- To maintain flexibility in your ITB, use your foam roller every day.

- If you overpronate, wear motion-control running shoes; if those alone don't work, try over-the-counter arch supports. I like heat-moldable orthotics, which you can find online.

- Increase your running cadence and shorten your stride. With a shorter stride, you will hit the ground closer to the center of your body mass, which improves your biomechanics for absorbing ground reaction forces. Count every time your feet strike the ground and aim for 170 to 180 strikes per minute.

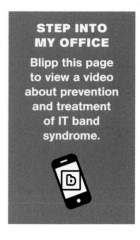

STEP INTO MY OFFICE

Blipp this page to view a video about prevention and treatment of IT band syndrome.

Arthritis of the Knee

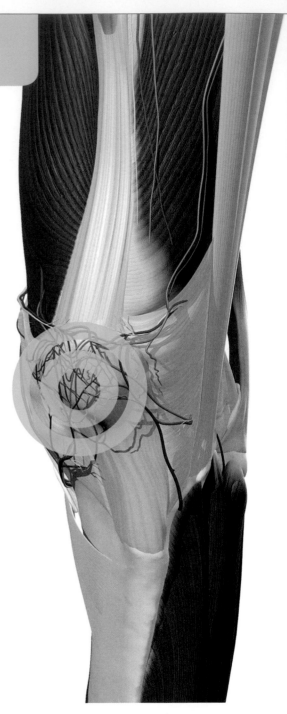

If you're over the age of 40, chances are you have had some aches and pains and have wondered about arthritis. The Latin roots *arthro* means joint and *itis* means inflammation. Arthritis is the chronic inflammation of a joint. Although arthritis can occur in any joint, runners most commonly get it in the ankles, knees, and hips.

I have had patients ask me, "Dr. Metzl, my friends tell me I'm going to get arthritis in my knees if I keep running. Is that true?" No—the knee is designed for forward leg motion. Arthritis happens for many reasons, including genetics, prior history of injury, or sometimes just bad luck. Whatever the reason, my focus as a running sports medicine doc is to try to make the symptoms as minimal as possible so you can stay on the road. Although this doesn't work in every runner, it's rare that I can't help someone using this approach. Let's have a look at arthritis so we can better understand how to both treat and prevent this common but very frustrating problem.

SYMPTOMS

- You will feel pain, swelling, and stiffness in your knee during running, walking, going up and down stairs, even getting up out of a chair—any activity that requires movement in the joint. Severe arthritis can seriously inhibit movement.

WHAT'S GOING ON

There are more than 100 types of arthritis, but the most common is osteoarthritis—the wearing out of hyaline cartilage (the lining of the joint), leaving bone to grind on bone.

Former injuries increase your risk of arthritis. If you have had an ACL tear, you are 50 percent more likely to develop arthritis in your knee. Genetics, overuse, and poor biomechanics also may play a role.

WHAT TO DO

Unfortunately, arthritis will worsen over time, but you can slow down the progression and, most importantly, you can continue to run. I have had patients with mild to moderate arthritis who are able to run successfully for years once we have made some of the modifications I suggest below.

- Keep moving. Research shows that regular activity is better than rest for keeping arthritic joints lubricated and slowing wear and tear. But focus more on low- or nonimpact activities such as swimming, cycling, and elliptical machines as you work on ways to alleviate pain. Cycling not only will offer the benefit of helping you maintain cardiovascular fitness but also will strengthen your legs to give more support to your knees.

- Take an anti-inflammatory, such as ibuprofen or naproxen, to help relieve pain and swelling.

- Viscosupplements are injections that lubricate the joint. These seem to offer temporary relief from arthritic knee pain, so ask your doc about them. Newer information suggests that platelet-rich plasma (PRP) injections might offer some relief as well (see page 36). The jury is still out, though, on the effectiveness of PRP for arthritis.

- Strengthen your quads, hips, and glutes. Strong quadriceps will take some of the load off your knees, which reduces pain and wear and tear. Strong muscles in the hips and butt will provide greater stability and help you run with improved mechanics, which also takes stress off your knees. See "Prevention" on page 86 for some of my favorite lower-body strengtheners.

- Overpronation puts more stress on the knees. If you are an overpronator, wear motion-control running shoes and consider over-the-counter arch supports.

- Check your stride length and cadence. Count every time your feet hit the ground for 1 minute. You want 170 to 180 footstrikes. A quicker cadence shortens your stride so your foot hits the ground closer to the center of your body mass. This improves your body's ability to absorb ground reaction forces as you run.

- Take your running to softer surfaces to lighten the impact. Asphalt is softer than concrete sidewalks; grass and dirt or cinder trails are softer still.

- If you think you have arthritis, see a sports physician, who will order an x-ray to confirm a diagnosis. She

85

should also do a full assessment of your strength, flexibility, and foot mechanics in addition to reviewing your running shoes, where you run, and your training. Since arthritis will worsen over time, it's best to see a doctor early to get a baseline of your condition against which you can measure its progression and evaluate how well treatment is working.

PREVENTION

I have one word for you—strength. A strong kinetic chain improves your stability during running; stability keeps your body in good alignment; and when your body is properly aligned, it does a better job of handling the stress of running. A strong kinetic chain can also take some of the load off your knees, and strong quads can be particularly helpful. Build up their strength to take on more of the work of running and your knees will thank you. (Instructions for the following exercises appear at the end of this chapter.)

- Do the IronStrength workout once or twice a week (see Chapter 12 and watch the videos).

- Use your foam roller daily to maintain loose muscles, and add 2 extra sets of the quad roll.

- Twice a week do the following exercises: prisoner squats, overhead dumbbell squats, dumbbell lunges, and low side-to-side lunges.

FOAM ROLLER EXERCISES

QUAD ROLLS

Lie facedown on the floor with your foam roller positioned above your right knee, supporting your upper body on bent arms. Cross your left leg over your right at the ankle. Roll your body back until the roller reaches the top of your thigh, and continue to move your quadriceps back and forth over the roller several times. Switch and roll your other quad. If it is too difficult to do this move with one leg over the other, lay with both of your thighs on the roller. Roll for 30 seconds.

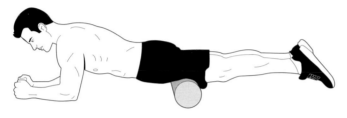

ITB ROLLS

Lie on your side on the floor with your foam roller under your leg beneath your hip. Support your upper body with your arm. Cross your left leg over your right and place your foot on the floor for support. Roll your leg from hip to knee over the roller, but do not roll onto the hip or knee joint. Do this at least once a day for 2 to 3 minutes on both legs.

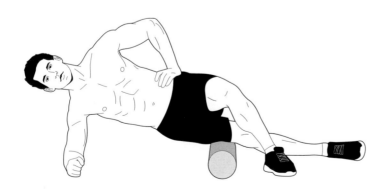

STRENGTH EXERCISES

STEP INSIDE THE GYM WITH ME

To watch a video showing how to do plyometric jump squats, turn to page 200.

PLYOMETRIC JUMP SQUATS

Stand tall with your feet a little more than shoulder-width apart and toes turned slightly outward. Put your arms straight out in front of you. Squat down, pushing your butt back while keeping your upper body tall. (If you can get your butt down below your knees, this move will give your glutes a good workout.) Now explode up as high as you can and land softly. Maintain a good anatomical position and keep the motion controlled, landing softly on your heels after each jump. Do 4 sets of 15.

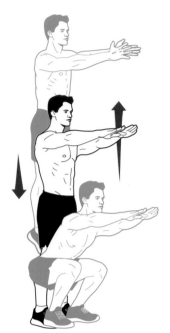

MOUNTAIN CLIMBERS

You can do these on the floor or use a bench or step. Get into a pushup position with your arms straight, shoulders over your hands, and legs straight behind you and supported on your toes. Bring your right knee straight into your chest, and then extend it straight back to the starting position. Then bring your left knee into your chest and back. Alternate your legs and move as fast as you can. As you do these, you want to maintain good form, keeping your back in a neutral position—not rounded, not drooping. The movement should come from your hips. Perform 3 sets of 15 reps, counting right and left together as 1 rep.

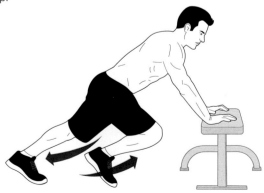

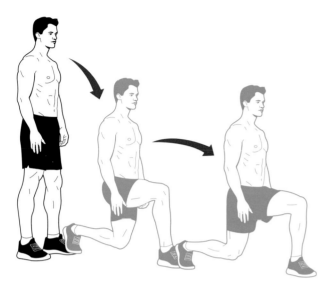

WALKING LUNGES (WITH OR WITHOUT DUMBBELLS)

Perform a lunge: From standing, bring your right leg forward and bend at the knee, lowering your back leg until it is parallel to the ground and your knee is almost touching the floor. Now instead of pushing back to the starting position, bring your back foot forward and swing it in front as if you were walking, lunging with that leg. Continue lunging forward, alternating legs. Do 3 sets of 15 reps, counting right and left together as 1 rep.

LEG EXTENSIONS

Sit in the leg extension machine with your legs under the padded bar, which should rest just above your ankles. Lift the weight by extending your legs straight out in front of you, and then slowly lower back to the starting position. You can also do this at home: Standing next to a chair for support, raise your leg, knee bent, until your thigh is parallel with the floor; then, keeping your thigh steady, slowly raise and drop your lower leg several times. It will seem easy at first, but after several reps you will feel the burn. Do 3 sets of 15 reps.

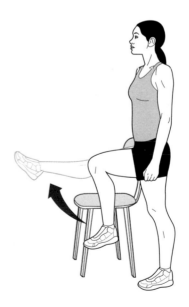

PLANKS

Get into a pushup position but bend your elbows and rest your weight on your forearms. Your body should form a straight line from your shoulders to your ankles. Engage your core, squeeze your glutes, and hold for 1 minute. Then roll to one side and hold your body up off the floor in a straight line from head to foot for 1 minute. Switch and do a plank on your other side.

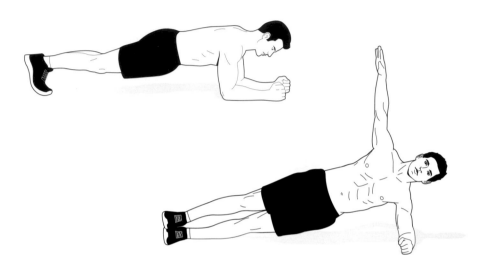

HIP RAISES

Lie on your back on the floor with your knees bent and feet flat on the floor. Squeezing your glutes, raise your hips until your body forms a straight line from your shoulders to your knees. Pause for 5 seconds, and then lower to the starting position. Do 3 sets of 15 reps daily.

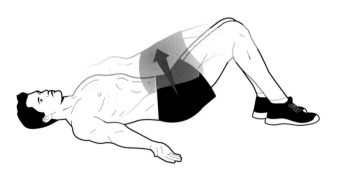

REVERSE HIP RAISES

Lie facedown on a bench with your torso on the bench and your hips off it. Keeping your legs nearly straight, lift them until they are in line with your torso. Squeeze your glutes, raise your hips, and pause; lower to the starting position. Do 3 sets of 15 reps daily.

Note: You can also do this exercise with a Swiss ball, placing your hands flat on the floor in front of you for support.

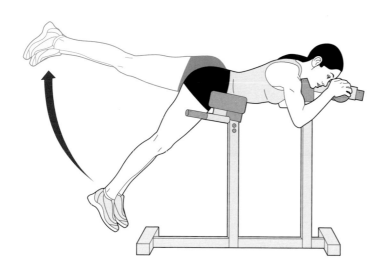

LOW SIDE-TO-SIDE LUNGES

Stand with your feet shoulder-width apart and facing straight ahead. Clasp your hands in front of your chest (or use dumbbells as illustrated). Shift your weight to your right leg and lower your body, bending your right knee and pushing your butt back. Keep your left leg straight and left foot flat on the floor. Without raising yourself all the way to standing, shift the movement to the left. Alternate back and forth for 15 reps on each side. Do a total of 3 sets daily. Be sure to push your hips back as you lower down and engage your core to keep your upper body vertical.

Challenge move: You can add dumbbells to this exercise. Hold them straight down in front of you with your palms facing in as you shift from one leg to the other.

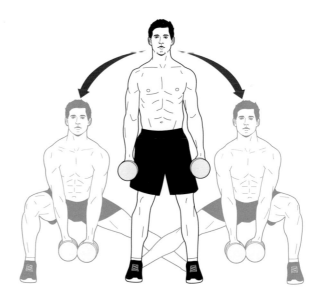

STANDING RESISTANCE-BAND HIP ABDUCTIONS

Secure a mini band to a sturdy object. Standing with your right leg next to the object, loop the band around your left ankle. Starting with your legs together, pull your left leg straight out to the side as far as you can, pause, and then return to the starting position. Do 15 reps and then switch sides. Complete 3 sets of 15 reps on each side daily.

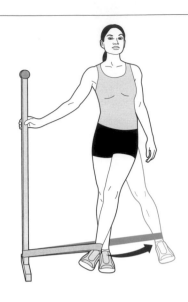

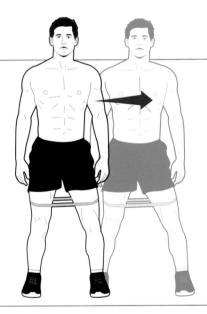

LATERAL BAND WALKS

Place a mini band around your legs just above your knees. Take small steps to your right for 20 feet, and then sidestep back to your left for 20 feet. As you do this exercise, keep your feet apart; don't bring them together. You want to maintain tension in the band. Do 3 sets daily.

PRISONER SQUATS

Stand tall with your feet shoulder-width apart. Put your hands behind your head (as if you have just been arrested) and pull your elbows and shoulders back. Lower your body, bending your knees and pushing your butt back as if you are going to sit down in a chair until you have reached a right angle at your knees. Pause, and then slowly push yourself back up to the starting position. Do 3 sets of 15 reps.

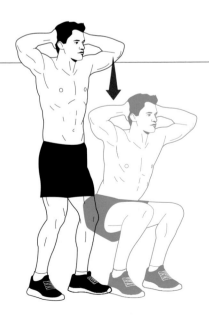

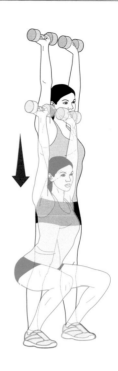

OVERHEAD DUMBBELL SQUATS

Stand with your feet slightly more than hip-width apart. Hold a pair of dumbbells and extend your arms straight up from your shoulders. Engage your core muscles and lower your body, bending your knees and pushing your butt back as if you are going to sit down in a chair. Go as deep as you can comfortably. Pause, and then slowly push yourself back up to the starting position. Keep your upper body as upright as possible, and don't let the dumbbells fall forward as you squat. Do 3 sets of 15 reps.

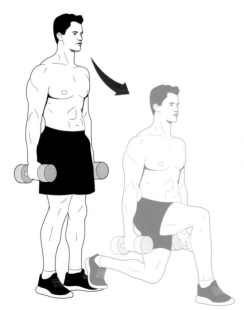

DUMBBELL LUNGES

Hold a pair of dumbbells straight down next to your sides, palms facing in. Engage your core, step forward with your right leg, and slowly lower your body until your back knee almost touches the ground and your front leg is bent about 90 degrees. Pause, and then push yourself back up to the starting position. Really use those core muscles to keep your upper body vertical. Do 15 reps, and then switch legs. Complete 3 sets with 15 reps on each side.

CHAPTER 7

YOUR UPPER LEGS

Your hamstrings and quadriceps are two of the biggest muscle groups in your body, and they perform two big jobs for runners: propulsion and stability.

Your hamstrings are biarticular, meaning they cross over two joints, the knee and hip. They bend your knee and also extend your hip as you push forward.

Your quad muscles all attach at the knee. They work opposite your hamstrings to extend your knee, and they help stabilize your knee during the stance, or landing, phase of running. Strong quads not only do a better job of keeping your knee stable but also can help ease the load on other stability muscles in your kinetic chain.

QUADRICEPS

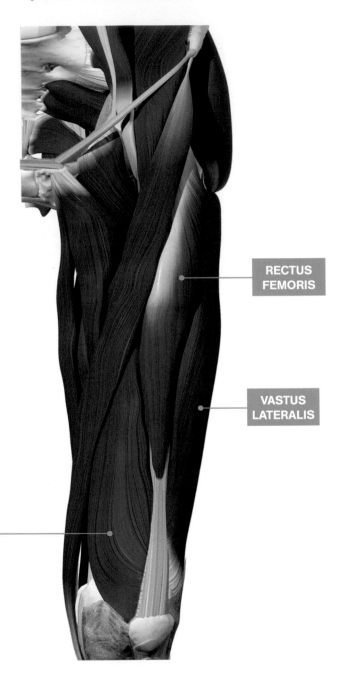

RECTUS FEMORIS

VASTUS LATERALIS

VASTUS MEDIALIS

HAMSTRINGS

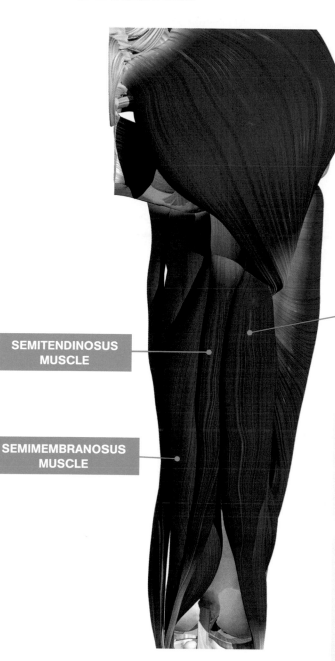

BICEPS
FEMORIS

SEMITENDINOSUS
MUSCLE

SEMIMEMBRANOSUS
MUSCLE

Where Does It Hurt?

1. If you feel anything from a twinge to a sharp pain in the front of your thigh as you're running, you probably have a *quad strain.*

2. Sudden, sharp pain in the middle of the back of your thigh as you're running signals a *middle-third hamstring strain.*

3. Pain high up in your hamstring or in your buttocks where the hamstring originates indicates a *proximal hamstring strain.*

Strained Quad

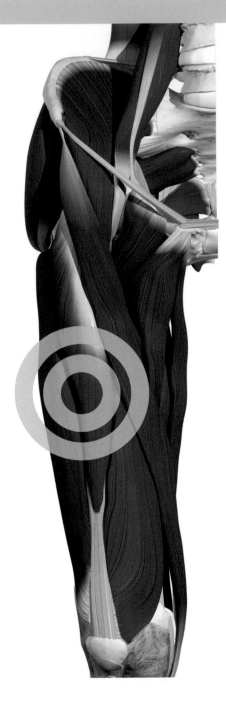

You're out running along, the sun is shining, the birds are chirping, you feel great. All of a sudden you change your stride to avoid a pothole in the road and—ouch!—you feel a slight tearing sensation in the front of your thigh. Welcome to the world of the quadriceps muscle strain.

SYMPTOMS

- Anything from a twinge to a sharp pain that occurs suddenly during a run
- A potential popping sensation when the strain occurred
- Tenderness, swelling, and bruising possible
- Pain when trying to straighten your leg against resistance
- Difficulty walking possible

WHAT'S GOING ON

Your muscle has been stretched farther than it can bear, and it tears. It's like pulling a piece of rope at both ends; as the strain increases, the fibers in the rope reach their breaking point and begin to tear. Quad strains generally occur during sprinting, when you ask for explosive power from this muscle group, and most often happen at the point where the muscle joins the tendon above the knee. Weak quadriceps are less able to withstand the stress and are vulnerable to strain, and tight quads are more easily torn.

WHAT TO DO

(Instructions for the stretches and exercises below appear at the end of this chapter.)

- Don't run or do anything that loads the muscle during the first 48 to 72 hours after the injury has occurred, depending on the severity of your strain. But do stay active; swimming, pool running, and the elliptical are all good options.

- Ice the painful area for 15 minutes four to six times a day for the first 2 days.

- If you have swelling, wrap it in a compression bandage and elevate your leg.

- Several days after you have strained your quad, try some gentle stretching. If you can do so comfortably, stretch your quad and hip flexors for 20 to 30 seconds four to six times a day with the quad stretch, hip flexor stretch, and kneeling hip flexor stretch.

- Three quad exercises work particularly well for rebuilding your injured muscles: straight-leg raises, simple lunges, and simple squats. As with stretching, you want to ease into them and do only as many repetitions as you can do comfortably. With time you will be able to do them more easily.

- If you are having difficulty walking or are not getting relief from the treatments described here, see a sports physician. She may order an MRI to determine the extent of your injury, and in addition to stretching and strengthening exercises, she may recommend ultrasound or electrostimulation treatment and sports massage.

PREVENTION

Strong, flexible muscles throughout your lower body will help prevent a strained quad. (Instructions for the exercises below appear at the end of this chapter.)

- Since you are most likely to strain your quad during quick, fast exertion, be sure to warm up with a mile or two of easy running before a speed workout or race. This will get your blood flowing, loosen up any tightness in your muscles, and prepare your body for the more intense running to come.

- Use your foam roller daily (see page 210).

- Add some hilly routes to your runs. Hill running is a great quad builder.

- Do the IronStrength workout once or twice a week (see Chapter 12 and watch the videos).

- Do reverse lunges with reach back, pistol squats, and split jumps daily as you rebuild strength, and twice a week to maintain it.

Strained or Pulled Hamstring (Middle Third)

A patient comes into my office and says, "I was running a 5-K and when I saw the finish line up ahead and realized I could get a PR, I started to go all out—and then it felt like someone stabbed me in the hamstring. I had to stop and limp to the finish." It's the classic story of a hamstring strain, or pull.

SYMPTOMS

- You will feel a sudden, sharp pain during a run that forces you to stop.
- You will feel pain when you apply pressure to your muscle with your hands.
- You will feel pain when you load your hamstring, which may be mild or excruciating depending on the severity of the strain.
- You may experience bruising or swelling.
- If you have injured your hamstring where it connects to the pelvis, you will feel the pain in your butt; this is called a proximal hamstring strain (see page 102 for details).

WHAT'S GOING ON

You have stretched your muscles farther than they can handle or have put a sudden and heavy load on them, or both. Let's take a look at what happens during sprinting. As you extend your leg forward, your hamstrings lengthen (or stretch), your foot hits the ground, and your hamstrings are loaded with both the force of your body weight hitting the ground and the load placed on your leg as you push your body forcefully forward. If your hamstring is weak or fatigued, or both, you have run into the perfect storm for a strain or pull.

Most hamstring strains occur in the muscle where it connects with the tendon down toward your knee, and most are mild and easily treated. In a severe grade 3 injury, the muscle is torn and will take months to heal.

WHAT TO DO

- As soon as possible after you have pulled your hamstring, ice it for 15 minutes, and continue to apply ice for 15 minutes four to six times a day for the first 2 days.

- Take a break from running, but use dynamic rest to maintain your conditioning. Swimming and cycling are good options here. Also, keep up with upper-body strengthening.

- A few days after the injury, you can begin gently performing the standing hamstring stretch and lying glutes stretch several times a day as shown at the end of this chapter.

- If you have torn or ruptured your hamstring, you will know it, and you will likely have seen your doctor before you opened this book. For a mild or moderate hamstring strain, if you are still in pain after 8 weeks, make an appointment with a sports physician. He may order an MRI or ultrasound to see what's going on in the muscle and then prescribe physical therapy and other treatments.

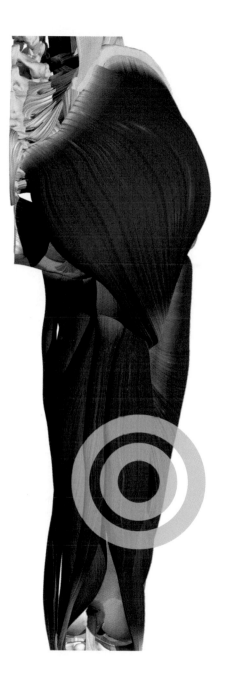

PREVENTION

I can't emphasize this enough: A strong kinetic chain is the key to a happy running life. You need to work your glutes, hip flexors, quads, and core as well as your hamstrings to prevent strains and tears. (Instructions for the exercises below appear at the end of this chapter.)

- Do the IronStrength workout once or twice a week (see Chapter 12 and watch the videos).

- Use your foam roller daily to prevent tightness (see page 210), and add 2 extra sets of the hamstring roll and the glute roll.

- Do the hip raise, the reverse hip raise, the walking lunge, planks, and the dumbbell stepup daily, especially as you return to running.

- Interval training, hill running, and stair climbing are other excellent activities for building hamstring strength.

Proximal Hamstring Strain (aka "the Pain in the Butt")

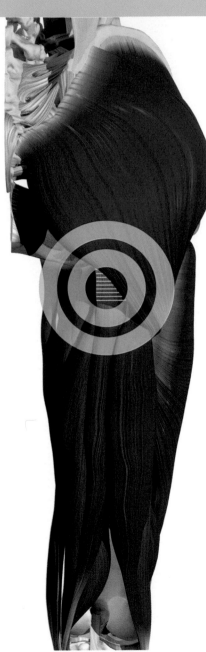

The issue here is that a quick strain or ache of the proximal hamstring can become a chronic pain in the butt in no time. Let's have a look and see how that happens.

SYMPTOMS

- You will experience aching pain during or after a run that is a real pain in the butt, sometimes bad enough to make you stop.

- You will feel pain that's especially uncomfortable during the push-off phase of running; the harder you push off, the worse it hurts, so speedwork and uphill running amplify the pain.

- You will feel pain from sitting on your "sit bones" throughout the day.

- It's easy to confuse piriformis syndrome with a proximal hamstring strain because both are pains in the butt. With piriformis syndrome, however, the pain comes from deep in your buttocks and may be accompanied by nerve pain that shoots down your hamstring. Sciatic nerve pain can also travel from the back into the buttock, so it's important to consider radiating pain from the back into the hip as a possible cause of butt pain as well. (See "Piriformis Syndrome" on page 129 for more information.)

WHAT'S GOING ON

Strains occur when you have overloaded your muscle and it actually begins to tear. In the case of a proximal hamstring strain, the injury occurs where the muscle connects to your tendon and attaches to your pelvis, at the ischial tuberosity—the bony part of your pelvis that you sit on. Since there is very little bloodflow in tendons, healing takes longer than with a strain to the muscle lower down in your hamstring. So do not ignore this pain.

WHAT TO DO

- As soon as you can after the injury has occurred, ice the area for 15 minutes, and continue to apply it for 15 minutes four to six times a day for the first 2 days.

- A few days after the injury, you can begin gently doing the standing hamstring stretch and the lying glutes stretch several times a day as shown at the end of this chapter.

- You may keep running on flat surfaces, but use a shorter stride. Shorten your stride by increasing your cadence. Count every time your right foot hits the ground for 1 minute and aim for 85 to 90 footstrikes.

- If your hamstring isn't getting better after 4 to 5 months of physical therapy and strength training, you may have a partial tear or chronic tendonosis. See your doctor. An MRI to aid diagnosis, followed by a platelet-rich plasma injection (see "PRP: Cutting-Edge Treatment" on page 36 for details) is a reasonable next step. An injection should only be considered if other avenues have been exhausted and if the area of pain correlates to changes on an MRI consistent with tendonosis or a chronic partial tear.

STEP INTO MY OFFICE

Blipp this page to view a video about the proximal hamstring strain, otherwise known as that pain in your butt.

PREVENTION

As I often say to my running patients, a strong butt is the key to a happy running life. There is nothing worse than a medical syndrome that I made up called weak butt syndrome. When your glutes are weak, more of the loading force of running is distributed along the proximal hamstring. And here's the chain of events that follows: Overload the proximal hamstring and you get tendonitis; over time tendonitis turns into tendonosis; eventually tendonosis can lead to a partial tear. By making the glutes strong, the loading forces of the hamstring are balanced out. Think of it like yin and yang. So keep those glutes strong, especially for hamstring health! (Instructions for the following exercises appear at the end of this chapter.)

- Do the IronStrength workout once or twice a week (see Chapter 12 and watch the videos). Really work those plyometric jump squats in the beginning, doing them daily.

- Do the split jumps and planks daily as you return to running.

- Use your foam roller daily to keep your muscles flexible (see page 210), and add 2 extra sets of the hamstring roll and the glute roll.

- Add speed workouts and hills into your running to build hamstring strength.

STRETCHES

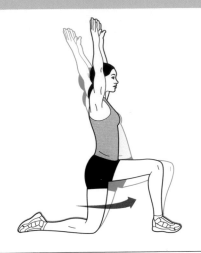

HIP FLEXOR STRETCHES

This move is part of the sun salutation from yoga. From standing, lower down and stretch your left leg back behind you, placing your knee on the floor. Your right leg should be bent at a 90-degree angle in front of you, foot flat on the floor. Push your hips forward as you raise your arms straight up and pull them back, arching your back just a little. Hold for 30 seconds, and then switch legs. Perform 3 sets.

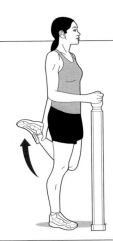

QUAD STRETCHES

Gentle at first! Stand on one leg near a wall or rail and grasping your other leg at the ankle, pull the ankle back and up toward your butt. Hold for 20 to 30 seconds, and then repeat with the other leg.

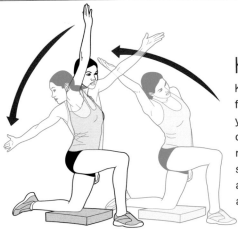

KNEELING HIP FLEXOR STRETCHES

Kneel down on your left knee and place your right leg in front of you, foot flat on the floor and knee bent 90 degrees. Reach straight up with your right hand as high as you can. Squeeze your glutes, engage your core, and bend to the right at your waist. Then rotate your torso to the right as you reach your right hand as far behind you as you can. You should feel the stretch in your left hip and quad. Hold for 30 seconds, and then switch sides. Do a total of 3 sets. Perform this stretch daily and up to three times a day if you are really tight.

STANDING HAMSTRING STRETCHES

Stand tall, extend your right leg straight out in front of you, and place your heel on a bench, step, or stable chair. Bend your left knee slightly and put your hands on your hips. Without rounding your back, bend at the hips toward your extended leg until you feel a gentle stretch in your hamstring. Hold for 30 seconds, and then switch sides. Repeat two more times on both legs. Perform this stretch up to three times a day if your hamstrings are really tight.

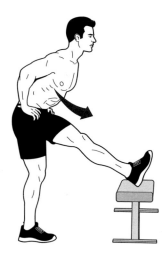

LYING GLUTES STRETCHES

Lie on your back on the floor, with your hips and knees bent so your calves are parallel to the floor. Cross your left leg over your right so your left ankle rests on your right thigh. Grasp your left knee with both hands and pull it toward the middle of your chest until you feel a gentle stretch in your glutes. Hold for 30 seconds, and then repeat on the other side. Repeat two more times on both legs. You can perform this stretch several times a day if your glutes are really tight.

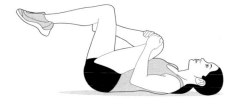

STRENGTH EXERCISES

STRAIGHT-LEG RAISES

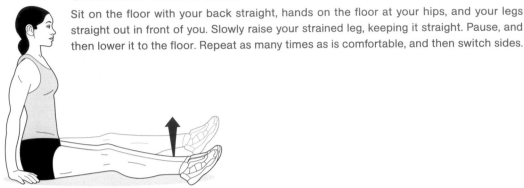

Sit on the floor with your back straight, hands on the floor at your hips, and your legs straight out in front of you. Slowly raise your strained leg, keeping it straight. Pause, and then lower it to the floor. Repeat as many times as is comfortable, and then switch sides.

CASE STUDY: KAYLA PHIPPS

Stats: Kayla is a 19-year-old college student who runs cross-country and track (200, 400, 800 meters) and has been a runner for 5 years.

Complaint: She pulled her left hamstring in high school and has had problems ever since. She didn't see a doctor and thought she would heal on her own—in her own words: "I thought I would be super-woman." Kayla kept running and thought she could continue to run, but her pain worsened.

Diagnosis: Kayla had tried everything to treat her injury: ice, heat, electrical stimulation, all in the context of many months of physical therapy. Despite her best efforts, she just wasn't getting any better and was becoming increasingly frustrated.

When I saw her, I looked through her information and her MRI, which showed no physical injury. This meant there wasn't anything anatomical that I needed to address, such as a partial tear. My assessment was that Kayla's pain was functional,

meaning her very strong hamstring muscles were actually too strong relative to her weaker glutes. My thought was that we needed to get her working on balancing her strength with a more aggressive plyometric-based strength program.

Treatment: I started Kayla on my IronStrength workout three times a week to build strength and prescribed daily use of a foam roller.

Outcome: One month after her initial visit, Kayla could run again. She still had some pain, but it did not interfere with her running biomechanics. Two months after that first meeting, Kayla was pain-free and still doing IronStrength workouts three times a week and foam rolling daily. Her running form is now more economical; she says her shoulder rotation is less pronounced. Her cardiovascular fitness has improved, and her race times are faster. Overall, just a huge win for Kayla and her hamstrings!

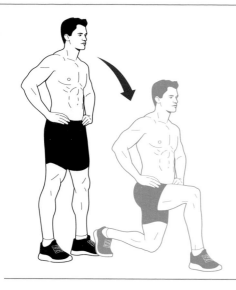

LUNGES

Stand tall, keeping your trunk upright and stable, and lunge forward with your right leg as you lower your body until your back knee nearly touches the ground. Pause, and then push yourself back to the starting position. Engage your core muscles to keep your upper body stable and upright; you don't want to bend forward or side to side. Complete 10 reps and switch sides, lunging with your left leg. Do 3 sets daily (1 set equals a right and left lunge).

SQUATS

Stand tall with your feet shoulder-width apart. With your arms straight out in front of you, lower your body, bending your knees and pushing your butt back as if you are going to sit down in a chair until you reach a right angle at your knees. Pause, and then slowly push yourself back up to the starting position. Do 15 reps and up to 3 sets daily.

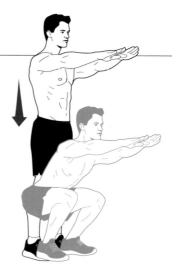

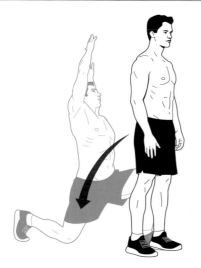

REVERSE LUNGES WITH REACH BACK

Stand tall with your arms straight down at your sides. Engage your core and lunge back with your right leg, lowering your body until your knee nearly touches the floor. As you lunge, reach your arms back over your shoulders and to the left. Return to the starting position and perform a total of 15 reps; then switch sides. Go for 3 sets of 15 reps on each side.

PLYOMETRIC LUNGES

From standing, step forward with your right leg, engage your core, and slowly lower your body as far as you can. Push up with enough force to switch your legs in the air so you land with your left foot forward. Engage your core muscles to keep your upper body vertical. Repeat, alternating legs for 3 sets of 15 reps; left and right together equals 1 rep.

Challenge move: Hold dumbbells at your sides as you perform the move.

HIP RAISES

Lie on your back on the floor with your knees bent and feet flat on the floor. Squeezing your glutes, raise your hips until your body forms a straight line from your shoulders to your knees. Pause for 5 seconds, and then lower to the starting position. Do 3 sets of 15 reps.

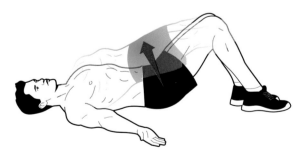

REVERSE HIP RAISES

Lie facedown on a bench with your torso on the bench and your hips off it. Keeping your legs nearly straight, lift them until they are in line with your torso. Squeeze your glutes, raise your hips, and pause; lower to the starting position. Do 3 sets of 15 reps.

Note: You can also do this exercise with a Swiss ball, placing your hands flat on the floor in front of you for support.

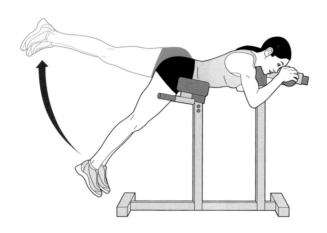

WALKING LUNGES (WITH OR WITHOUT DUMBBELLS)

Perform a lunge: From standing, bring your right leg forward and bend at the knee, lowering your back leg until it is parallel to the ground and your knee is almost touching the floor. Now, instead of pushing back to the starting position, bring your back foot forward and swing it in front as if you were walking, lunging with that leg. Continue lunging forward, alternating legs, for a total of 15 repetitions, counting right and left together as 1 rep. Do 3 sets of reps.

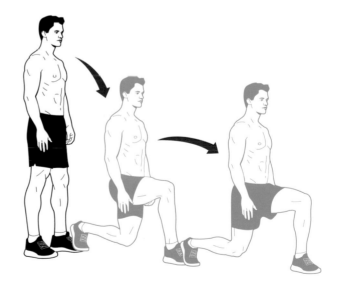

PLANKS

Get into a pushup position but bend your elbows and rest your weight on your forearms. Your body should form a straight line from your shoulders to your ankles. Engage your core, squeeze your glutes, and hold for 1 minute. Then roll to one side and hold your body up off the floor in a straight line from head to foot for 1 minute. Switch and do a plank on your other side.

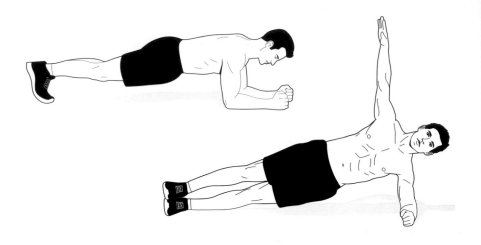

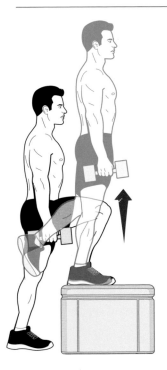

DUMBBELL STEPUPS

Hold a pair of dumbbells straight down at your sides. Stand in front of a bench or step and plant your right foot firmly on it (the bench or step should be at a height that produces a 90-degree bend at your knee). Using your heel, push your body up onto the step until you are standing straight on your right leg with your left leg elevated behind you. Lower down until your left foot touches the floor. Engage your core muscles to keep your upper body vertical as you do this move. Perform 15 reps with your right leg, and then switch sides. Do 3 sets of 15 reps on each side.

CHAPTER 8

YOUR HIPS, GROIN, AND GLUTES

If there's one phrase you will hear over and over from me, it's this: A strong butt is key to a happy running life.

Strong glutes provide stability, maintain a level pelvis, and power your running. The largest group of muscles in your body, they work together with your core, hips, and hamstrings to keep you in good alignment for injury-free running. Maintain strength and flexibility in all of these muscles and you will be one very happy runner!

Where Does It Hurt?

Hip pain, groin pain—it's easy to confuse the two. Here's the key difference: You will feel the pain of a hip injury either in the side of your hip or in the front at the hip joint; groin injuries present themselves at or around your pubic bone near the midline of your body.

Hips

1. If you feel pain on the outside of your hip along the bony prominence at the top of your thigh bone, you are looking at *bursitis.*

2. Pain in the front of the hip at the hip joint during running is a sign of a *stress fracture* or a *hip flexor strain.* To differentiate between the two, do the hop test—hop up and down on your injured side. If it hurts when you land, you probably have a stress fracture.

Groin

1. If you feel pain in your inner thigh at your groin when you bring your legs together, that's a sign of a *sports hernia,* or *adductor strain.* It will hurt during and after running.

2. A *stress injury or fracture* to the femoral neck or the pubic ramus portion of your pelvic bone is really painful. It hurts when you land during running and when you do the hop test.

3. *Osteitis pubis* is chronic inflammation caused by the rubbing together of the two major bones of the pelvis where they come together in the front. It hurts a lot, and you will feel the pain right at the center of your groin. A distinguishing characteristic: It tends to hurt when you cross your legs while seated or standing.

Glutes

A pain in the butt may not mean an injury to the butt; a problem in your hamstrings or lower back could be the source. Let's use my pain-in-the-butt flowchart to figure out what's going on.

1. Pain that's low, where your glutes meet your hamstrings, indicates a *proximal hamstring strain* (see page 102 for details).

2. Pain more centrally located in your butt could mean a strained glute, piriformis syndrome, or sciatica.

    a. If the discomfort is contained in your glutes and there is no radiating pain, you most likely have a *strained glute.*

    b. If you experience shooting pain down your legs or into your lower back along with discomfort in your butt, you are looking at *piriformis syndrome* or *sciatica*. To differentiate here, piriformis syndrome is a pinching of the sciatic nerve at the piriformis muscle deep in the gluteal region. The nerve can also be pinched higher, at the level of the spine, in which case the pain radiates from the spine down to the butt. That's why butt pain is often best evaluated by a sports doc if the first line of treatments I suggest don't help right away.

    i. If the primary pain comes from deep within your butt on one side and worsens when you sit down, you likely have *piriformis syndrome.* Any associated shooting pains travel down the back of your leg and only go as far as your hamstring.

    ii. *Sciatic pain* sits primarily in your lower back, and shooting pain may travel down the back of one or both of your legs and can reach as far as your toes (see pages 145–146 for how to treat and prevent sciatica).

Though I have delineated the specific pain characteristics of these different injuries, the truth is, in real life the lines are often blurry, even for sports docs. If a patient is experiencing a lot of pain in the pubic area or the front of the hip, I will order an MRI to confirm a diagnosis. And in the case of stress fractures of the femoral neck and the pubic ramus, again, an MRI is needed to determine which one is present (see "Stress Fracture" on page 119 for more information). Let's look at how to make sense of all these different aches and pains and how to fix them.

STEP INTO MY OFFICE

Blipp this page to view a video about prevention and treatment of various hip injuries.

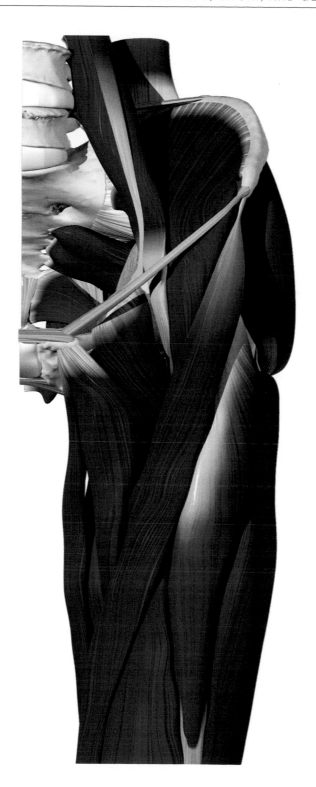

Bursitis

If you're a side sleeper and your hip wakes you up at night, the cushioning in your hip might be to blame.

SYMPTOMS

- You will feel pain on the outside of your hip, particularly at the point where the bony area at the top of your thigh bone—called the greater trochanter—protrudes. It may feel sharp and intense at first and then turn into achiness that you feel during and after running.

- The pain may intensify when you get up out of a chair or go up stairs.

- You will experience discomfort when you are lying on your injured side.

WHAT'S GOING ON

Lying next to the greater trochanter is a fluid-filled sac called a bursa. You have several bursae in your body, and their job is to create cushioning between bones and soft tissue (muscles and tendons) to reduce friction. The bursa at the greater trochanter comes between the bone and a small muscle called the tensor fascia latae (TFL), which farther down your leg joins the iliotibial band (ITB, a band of tissue that runs down along the outside of your thigh). A tight TFL squeezes the bursa against the bone, and the result is inflammation and pain. Let's look at a few possible causes.

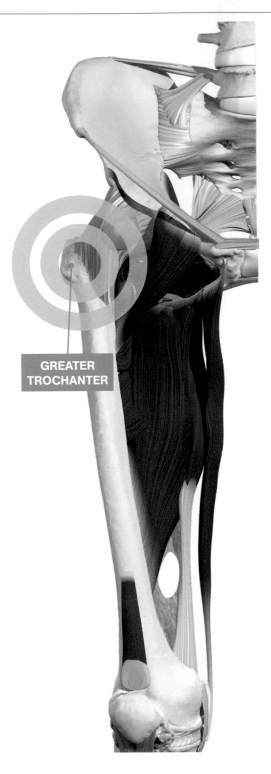

GREATER
TROCHANTER

- If you have weak muscles in your hips, you will have less stability in your hips and more motion as you run, which creates greater tension in the ITB and TFL and squeezes the bursa. Over lots of miles, this leads to inflammation.

- Overpronation—when the foot rolls too far inward during running— also increases tension along the outside of your leg.

- Bursitis can result from simple tightness along the ITB and TFL.

WHAT TO DO

- If your pain is mild and doesn't affect your form, you may keep running, but if you find that you are favoring that hip and changing your biomechanics in any way, switch to cardio that you can do comfortably and continue with strength exercises as you are able.

- Ice the sore area for 15 minutes four to six times a day for the first 2 days.

- Take an anti-inflammatory, such as ibuprofen or naproxen, to reduce pain and swelling.

- Wear shoes with good medial support to help limit pronation, or try over-the-counter orthotics. My

favorites: heat-moldable inserts. Search for them online.

- If you can do so without too much pain, stretch the ITB and TFL as shown at the end of this chapter.

- As the pain eases up, begin strengthening your core and the muscles around your hips using the Iron-Strength workout once or twice a week (see Chapter 12 and watch the videos).

- Bursitis should clear up with a little TLC, but if you still have pain after 3 weeks, see your sports physician, who may recommend a cortisone injection into the bursa to shrink it.

PREVENTION

A strong core and strong muscles around your hips create greater stability when you run, resulting in less tension along the ITB and TFL.

- Perform the IronStrength workout once or twice a week (see Chapter 12 and watch the videos).

- Keep the TFL and ITB flexible by using your foam roller every day (see page 210), and add 2 extra sets of the ITB rolls (see page 87).

CASE STUDY: REBECCA GUENTHER

Stats: Rebecca is a 61-year-old librarian who has been running for 33 years.

Complaint: She was experiencing soreness on the outside of her left hip. She used ice and ibuprofen and took a break from running but found the hip was still painful when she tried running again.

Diagnosis: X-rays and an MRI showed everything was normal, so I sent Rebecca for a running analysis to find out what biomechanical issues she might be having. Overall, I was pretty happy with Rebecca's results, but they did reveal that her left glute was weak, and there was an imbalance between the glute and the muscles on the outside of her left hip—nothing dramatic, but enough to create strain across her tensor fascia latae (TFL), a small muscle at the hip that connects to the iliotibial band. In addition, a treadmill analysis showed Rebecca was overstriding just a bit.

Treatment: I prescribed the IronStrength workout, which she started immediately after our first visit, and our physical therapist gave her a few additional exercises. I also advised her to shorten her stride by boosting her cadence to 85 to 90 strides a minute.

Outcome: One month after our initial visit, Rebecca was running pain-free and had signed up for a half-marathon.

Hip Flexor Tendonitis

The hip flexors (aka iliopsoas) include the psoas and iliacus muscles. They originate at the vertebrae in your lower back, run down through the pelvis, and attach on the inner side of the femur. They are big muscles, and they have two main jobs: to help you bend forward at the waist and to help you pull your knee up toward your chest.

SYMPTOMS

Pain in the front of the hip can be caused by tendonitis or a stress fracture. To differentiate between the two, do the hop test: Hop up and down a couple times on your injured side. If it hurts when you land, that's a stress fracture. It's important to know that in first-time marathoners, what is sometimes thought to be a hip flexor strain is actually a hip stress fracture. If the hop test is painful, your doc should be concerned about a stress fracture in the pubic symphysis or femoral neck. These diagnoses can be really tricky, so if it hurts, be safe and get it checked out before it gets worse!

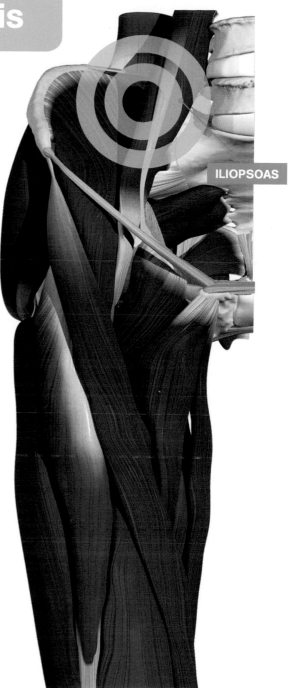

ILIOPSOAS

WHAT'S GOING ON

Tendonitis is an overuse injury, occurring when you run more miles than your muscle is prepared to handle. Too much uphill running, which requires you to pull your knee up higher than flat running, is particularly hard on your hip flexors. Also, if your muscles are tight, they are more easily strained.

Tight hip flexors have other consequences too. They tilt your pelvis, and a tilted pelvis can lead to lower-back problems. They also mess with your biomechanics and set you up for possible knee injuries. So you have lots of reasons to keep these muscles flexible.

WHAT TO DO

- Apply ice to the sore area for 15 minutes four to six times a day for 2 days.

- Take an anti-inflammatory, such as ibuprofen or naproxen, to ease the pain and reduce swelling.

- Do not run or engage in any activity that requires you to raise your knee. Try swimming, and if it feels comfortable, go with it. Continue with upper-body strength training.

- Gently stretch your muscles using the hip flexor stretch and the piriformis stretch shown at the end of this chapter.

- A hip flexor strain should heal in 2 to 8 weeks, but if it persists beyond that, make an appointment with a sports doc, who may order an MRI or ultrasound to see exactly what's going on before prescribing a treatment plan.

PREVENTION

Your hip flexors work with your core muscles, glutes, quadriceps, and hamstrings, so it's important to strengthen all of these muscles and maintain their flexibility.

- Do the IronStrength workout once or twice a week (see Chapter 12 and watch the videos).

- Stay flexible by using your foam roller every day (see page 210).

- Twice a week, do the following exercises: mountain climbers, plyometric jump squats, reverse lunges with reach back, planks, and the Swiss ball pike, all shown at the end of this chapter.

Stress Fracture (of the Hip and Pelvis)

As I discussed for the foot and shin, stress fractures are nasty injuries that can get worse quickly. Stress fractures in the hip are particularly common among first-time marathoners and can take many months to heal. The discussion here applies to both fractures of the femoral neck (where the femur, or thigh bone, meets your pelvis) and fractures of the pelvic bone.

SYMPTOMS

- You will feel pain in the front of your hip when you land during running.

- Do the hop test: Hop straight up and down a few times on your injured leg. If it hurts when you land, chances are you have a stress injury or fracture.

WHAT'S GOING ON

A classic overuse injury, stress fractures occur when the load to the bone is greater than it can bear. If you continue to run on a stressed bone, it swells and over time cracks. There are several factors that can contribute.

- Upping your mileage too fast, which doesn't give your bone time to get stronger in response to the stresses of running

- Always running on asphalt or, worse, concrete

- Overstriding or lack of stability in your hips, which puts extra stress on the joint

- Finally, low bone density caused by poor nutrition or, in women, amenorrhea, which makes bones more fragile

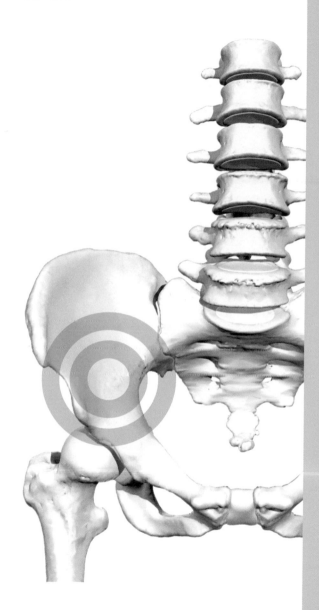

WHAT TO DO

- See your doctor as soon as you suspect a stress fracture. He will order an x-ray and/or an MRI. A stress fracture will only show up on an x-ray, however, if it is very serious and the bone is cracking or when it is beginning to heal. After confirming a diagnosis, your doctor will work with you to determine the cause of the stress fracture and then a plan for recovery.

- Absolutely no running or any weight-bearing activity while recovering from a stress fracture. Swim, cycle, run in the pool, or use the elliptical to maintain fitness as you heal. And keep up with upper-body strength training. Be sure to consult with your doctor and physical therapist before you return to running.

- If you have a family history of osteoporosis or you are a woman and experiencing amenorrhea, your physician may order a bone density test. This may lead to a comprehensive strategy to improve bone density that includes nutrition, strength training, and sometimes even oral contraceptive pills. The key here is that the diagnosis of a stress fracture is only half the battle; the main issue is to figure out why it's happening so you can prevent future problems.

- When you are pain-free, begin doing squats and multidirectional lunges (shown at the end of this chapter) twice a week. Don't do any high-impact moves until your doctor gives you the okay. In general, I have my patients build strength and then gradually increase mileage. When they have been running pain-free for a month, I will start adding in speed work.

PREVENTION

Strong muscles in your butt, core, hips, and legs will support your hips during running and prevent excess strain on the hip joints.

- Do the IronStrength workout once or twice a week (see Chapter 12 and watch the videos).

- Keep muscles flexible by using your foam roller daily (see page 210).

- Be sure to follow the 10 percent rule: Don't increase mileage by more than 10 percent from week to week.

- A shorter, quicker stride can reduce stress on you hip joint. On your next run, count every time your right foot hits the ground for 60 seconds. You want a number between 85 and 90.

- Never run on concrete surfaces. Asphalt, though hard, has some give. And a cinder path, a well-groomed trail, or a track is even easier on your body.

- Make sure you get enough calcium and vitamin D daily: 1,000 milligrams of calcium (women over 50 and men over 70 need 1,200 milligrams); 600 IU of vitamin D (all adults over 70 need 800 IU). The best sources are dairy products (see Chapter 15 for other options).

CASE STUDY: JILL MYERS

Stats: Jill is a 39-year-old mom of two boys and has been a runner for 5 years.

Complaint: Jill was experiencing pain in her groin. She explained that it started out as dull pain that worsened as she ran. Her running partner had a groin pull with similar symptoms, so Jill assumed she had the same and treated it with stretching. She continued running, and after a few weeks the pain stabbed her like a knife. Jill said it felt like something was pulling apart in her groin.

Diagnosis: Suspecting a stress fracture, I asked Jill to do the hop test, which was very painful, so I then ordered an MRI, which confirmed a fracture in the pubic ramus. She had no family history of osteoporosis. The cause of her stress fracture was biomechanical: She had very weak core muscles and wasn't able to effectively support her pelvis during landing. Also, she was overstriding. The end result was too much stress on her pelvic bones.

Treatment: I advised Jill not to run but gave her the green light to walk. Two months after her diagnosis, the bone had healed and I started her on the Iron-Strength workouts. Treatment for stress fractures happens in phases. In phase one, I let the bone heal while encouraging my patients to cross-train to maintain fitness. As the bone heals, I address the reasons the injury happened. In Jill's case, the issue wasn't a lack of bone density but a lack of strength—a biomechanical injury. Once the bone healed, I helped her fix the reasons the injury happened in the first place to prevent recurrence. Phase three: a gradual return to running.

Outcome: Jill achieved a 100 percent recovery and today is running healthy and pain-free.

Sports Hernia (aka Adductor Strain or Tear/Groin Strain)

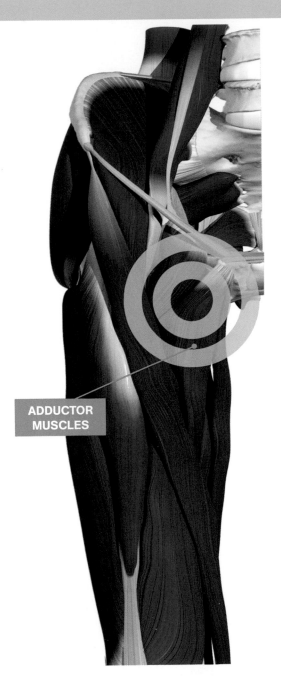

ADDUCTOR MUSCLES

Not to be confused with the common abdominal version, this hernia is a strain of the adductor muscle along your inner thigh, where it attaches to the pelvic bone.

SYMPTOMS

- You will feel pain at the top of your inner thigh where it meets your pubic bone. A minor strain sends out dull pain that gets worse over time; a sudden pull or tear busts out a sharp pain.

- It's possible to confuse a sports hernia with other injuries—a strained hip flexor, for example. Move the knee of your injured leg toward your other leg as you create resistance by pushing against the injured leg; if you feel pain up inside your inner thigh at the groin, then you're looking at a sports hernia.

- You may experience swelling.

WHAT'S GOING ON

The adductors are a group of muscles that originate at the pelvic bone and attach to the femur (the thigh bone) on the inside of your leg. They bring your leg in toward the centerline of your body and help to stabilize your hip as you run.

Sudden acceleration, like when you're sprinting for the finish line of a race or when you're running fast intervals, can overload weak or inflexible muscles and cause a strain or tear, usually at the point where the muscle attaches to the pelvic bone.

WHAT TO DO

(Instructions for the stretches and exercises below appear at the end of this chapter.)

- Ice the area for 15 minutes as soon as possible after the injury, and then continue to apply ice for 15 minutes four to six times a day for the first 2 days.

- If you have swelling and inflammation, try an anti-inflammatory, such as ibuprofen or naproxen.

- If mild pain doesn't affect your mechanics, you can continue to run as you treat the strain, but if you find that you're altering your running form in any way, use dynamic rest—swim, bike, whatever doesn't hurt—to maintain your cardiovascular fitness. And keep up with your upper-body strength work.

- Stretch the area gently when you can do so with little to no pain; use the sitting and standing groin stretches.

- Strengthen your adductors by doing low side-to-side lunges and diagonal lunges when you can do these exercises comfortably.

Because there is very little bloodflow in this area, this injury can take a long time to heal.

STEP INTO MY OFFICE

Blipp this page to view a video about prevention and treatment of groin injuries.

CASE STUDY: JEFF DENGATE

Stats: Jeff is a 37-year-old elite-level competitive distance runner and member of Central Park Track Club.

Complaint: Jeff had pain deep in his groin, but as many runners do, he continued to run with that pain for 18 months. And then it became significantly worse. He said it felt like someone was stabbing him.

Diagnosis: I had Jeff do the one-legged hop test, in which you jump a few times on your injured side, and he felt okay, so I was pretty sure he didn't have a stress fracture. But I ordered an MRI to confirm, and it came back negative. During that same initial visit, I had Jeff try some single-leg squats, and his performance was pretty abysmal. So I asked the question I ask all my runners: "Do you do any strength training?" And the answer I got was the same one I hear from most of the runners who come see me: "No." The diagnosis was clear—a sports hernia, resulting from weak glutes and hip muscles.

Treatment: I prescribed the IronStrength workout, which Jeff began immediately and enthusiastically and continues to do today.

Outcome: Jeff achieved 100 percent recovery and is now a big fan of IronStrength.

- If you have difficulty bringing the knee on your injured side close to the other knee, you may have a severe tear or rupture. See your sports physician. She will order an MRI or ultrasound to see what the damage is and then prescribe treatment. If your injury persists, your doctor may recommend platelet-rich plasma injections ("PRP: Cutting-Edge Treatment" on page 36 to learn more).

PREVENTION

The best way to prevent a sports hernia is through strength training.

- Do the IronStrength workout once or twice a week (see Chapter 12 and watch the videos).

- Do low side-to-side lunges, diagonal lunges, plyometric jump squats, and skaters (shown at the end of this chapter) daily.

Osteitis Pubis

Remember the cartoons in which the characters would rub two sticks together to make a fire? (I guess you can do that in real life too, but I was never successful.) Well, that's kind of how this injury happens. Only the two sticks are the bones in your pelvis. If you're thinking "Ouch!" you're right.

SYMPTOMS

- You will feel pain in the middle of your groin right around the centerline of your body that hurts all the time.

WHAT'S GOING ON

The two major bones of your pelvis come together at a cartilaginous joint called the pubic symphysis. When the bones rub together, inflammation occurs. I see this injury often among

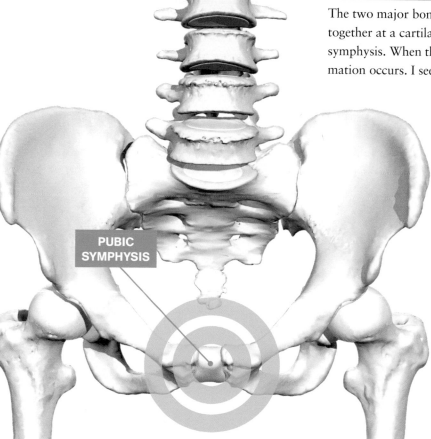

PUBIC SYMPHYSIS

women who start running too quickly after pregnancy. During pregnancy, a woman's body produces the hormone relaxin, which loosens the symphysis to allow the baby to pass through. After the baby is born, while the area is still relaxed, it is more vulnerable to injury.

An imbalance between your abdominal muscles and adductors (muscles that originate at the pelvic bone and attach to the femur), which help stabilize your pelvis during running, can also lead to osteitis pubis.

WHAT TO DO

(Instructions for the stretches and exercises below appear at the end of this chapter.)

- Sorry, no running or any other activity that causes pain. Try cycling, pool running, or swimming to maintain your cardio fitness. If you treat this injury early, recovery can take anywhere from 3 to 8 weeks. Run through the pain and you may end up sidelined for months.

- Take an anti-inflammatory, such as ibuprofen or naproxen, to reduce the pain.

- Ice the area for 15 minutes four to six times a day.

- Stretch your adductor muscles using the sitting and standing groin stretches.

- Strengthen your adductors by doing low side-to-side lunges and diagonal lunges when you can do them with little to no pain.

- If after 3 weeks of home treatment your pain isn't getting any better, see a sports physician. He will order an x-ray and possibly an MRI to confirm osteitis pubis and then recommend treatment. Your doc may also suggest a cortisone injection directly into the symphysis, which clears up the inflammation in most cases.

PREVENTION

The best way to prevent groin strains is to build strength in your adductors and your core (the adductors and core muscles work together).

- Do the IronStrength workout once or twice a week (see Chapter 12 and watch the videos).

- Do low side-to-side lunges, diagonal lunges, plyometric jump squats, and skaters (all shown at the end of this chapter) daily.

Strained Glute

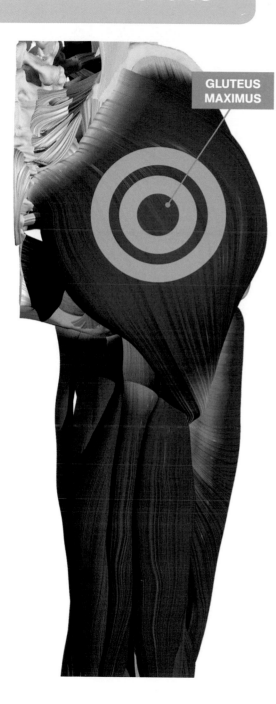

GLUTEUS MAXIMUS

Your glutes are a group of three muscles: the gluteus maximus, gluteus medius, and gluteus minimus. They attach to your pelvic bone and your femur and provide stability and power as you run.

SYMPTOMS

- A sharp pain or pulling in your glutes
- In mild cases, pain that doesn't interfere with your running but can be felt when you stop
- In more severe strains, pain while you run as well as afterward, and possible pain when you go up and down stairs, walk uphill, or even sit down

WHAT'S GOING ON

Strains commonly occur when the muscle contracts during a lengthening phase of activity, such as when you suddenly accelerate during running. Think about it: You are extending your leg—lengthening the muscles in your glutes—but the suddenness and quickness of the movement causes your muscle to respond with contraction. Essentially your muscle is being "pulled" in opposite directions at the same time. Ouch!

WHAT TO DO

- Ice the painful area for 15 minutes four to six times a day for 2 days.
- You may continue to run as long as pain doesn't interfere with your mechanics. When or if it does, switch to swimming or another

cardio activity that you can do without pain.

- Continue to strength-train, but don't do any moves that involve jumping or lunging. Also, avoid stairs whenever possible.

- Try an anti-inflammatory, such as ibuprofen or naproxen, to ease the pain and inflammation.

- When you can do so without too much discomfort, perform the following moves daily: the glute roll, the lying glutes stretch, the gluteal bridge, and chair squats (all shown at the end of this chapter). Start slowly, gradually increasing your effort until you can do a set of 10 to 20 reps three times a day.

- If pain is severe or you haven't recovered after about 6 weeks, see your doctor.

PREVENTION

Not only is it important to keep your butt strong, but you also need to strengthen the muscles in your core, hips, and hamstrings. Weakness in one or more of these areas can affect the performance of your glutes and lead to injury.

- Do the IronStrength workout once or twice a week (see Chapter 12 and watch the videos).

- Perform plyometric jump squats, planks, burpees, and the dumbbell split squats (all shown at the end of this chapter) daily.

- Build your hamstrings and glutes on the run by including intervals, hills, or hill sprints.

- Use your foam roller daily to keep muscles flexible and work out any tight spots (see page 210).

Piriformis Syndrome

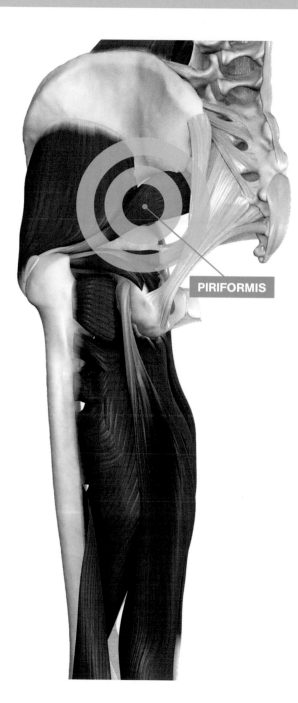

PIRIFORMIS

The piriformis is a small muscle that lies deep within your buttocks and right next to the sciatic nerve. Its role in running is to help stabilize your hip as you land. As small as this muscle is, it can cause a big problem.

SYMPTOMS

- You will have pain that originates deep in your butt but may shoot down your hamstring or up into your lower back.

- Sitting or putting pressure on your butt will be especially painful.

- The pain of piriformis syndrome is very similar to sciatic pain (see page 145), and with good reason—in both cases a pinched sciatic nerve is the cause. If you have piriformis syndrome, however, the pain comes from deep within your glutes on one side and is worse when you sit. Also, if you experience shooting pain with piriformis syndrome, it doesn't travel farther than your hamstrings—again on one side. Sciatic shooting pains can travel down both legs and even reach your toes.

WHAT'S GOING ON

The piriformis muscle originates at the base of your spine and attaches to your femur (thigh bone). It lies on top of your sciatic nerve, so when the piriformis becomes too tight, it squeezes the sciatic nerve, causing pain. Piriformis pain can also come from the spine, where a pinched nerve in the back radiates pain down into the butt, often masquerading as a piriformis

STEP INTO MY OFFICE

Blipp this page to view a video about two common pains in the butt: proximal hamstring strain and piriformis syndrome.

problem. A doctor and a back MRI can help diagnose this if the symptoms persist.

Why does your piriformis become tight? Remember your kinetic chain: Your piriformis works with your glutes, hamstrings, and hip muscles, and weakness in one or more of those muscles puts extra strain on the piri-

formis, which then tightens up and squeezes the sciatic nerve.

Also, if you overpronate, as your foot rolls inward it causes your knee to rotate. One of the jobs of the piriformis is to help prevent your knee from rotating too much. Over time too much pronation creates too much rotation and tension along the piriformis.

WHAT TO DO

(Instructions for the stretches and glute roll below appear at the end of this chapter.)

- You may keep running, but if the pain alters your running mechanics in any way, find a cardio activity that doesn't hurt and continue with upper-body strengthening.

- Take an anti-inflammatory, such as ibuprofen or naproxen, to ease the pain. This will allow you to comfortably stretch and roll the muscle.

- Stretch your piriformis muscle daily

with the piriformis stretch and the pigeon stretch.

- Use your foam roller every day to roll your glutes and relax the muscle around the nerve.

- If you don't feel better in a week, see your doctor to confirm a diagnosis. She may simply recommend that you continue with home treatment or prescribe muscle relaxants. If conservative treatments fail, your doc may suggest an injection of an anesthetic or cortisone.

PREVENTION

- Do the IronStrength workout once or twice a week (see Chapter 12 and watch the videos).

- Every day perform the standing resistance-band hip abduction, lateral band walks, plyometric jump squats, planks, and fire hydrant in-out (all shown at the end of this chapter).

- Use your foam roller every day to keep muscles loose and work out any tight spots (see page 133).

- Wear a motion-control shoe to prevent overpronation; if that doesn't help, try over-the-counter inserts.

STRETCHES

ITB/TFL STRETCHES

Lie on your back on the floor and lift the leg on your painful side straight up in the air. Slowly bring that leg across your body and lower it as far as you can. Hold for 15 seconds, and then raise your leg back to vertical. Do 3 to 5 reps.

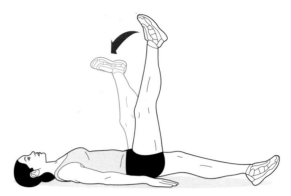

HIP FLEXOR STRETCHES

This move is part of the sun salutation from yoga. From standing, lower down and stretch your left leg back behind you, placing your knee on the floor. Your right leg should be bent at a 90-degree angle in front of you, foot flat on the floor. Push your hips forward as you raise your arms straight up and pull them back, arching your back just a little. Hold for 30 seconds, and then switch legs. Perform 3 sets.

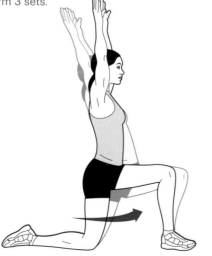

PIRIFORMIS STRETCHES

Lie on your back, knees bent and feet flat on the floor. Bring your right leg up, cross it over your left leg, and rest your ankle against your thigh. Maintaining this position, pull your left leg in toward your chest. Hold for 20 to 30 seconds, and repeat two more times. Then switch sides.

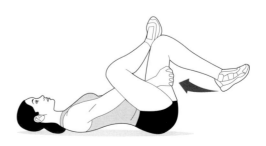

SITTING GROIN STRETCHES

Sit on the floor with your knees bent to the sides and the bottoms of your feet pressed together. Using your elbows, gently push the tops of your knees toward the floor. Pause and hold for 10 to 15 seconds, and then release. Repeat three to five times.

STANDING GROIN STRETCHES

Stand with your feet shoulder-width apart. Shift your weight to one side, bending your knee slightly and pausing when you feel the stretch in your inner thigh. Hold for 10 to 15 seconds, and then return to the starting position. Repeat three to five times; then stretch the other side.

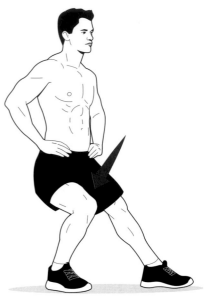

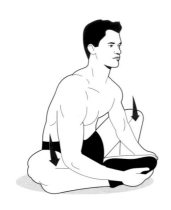

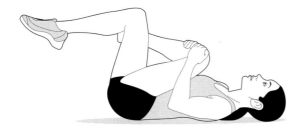

LYING GLUTES STRETCHES

Lie on your back on the floor, with your hips and knees bent so your calves are parallel to the floor. Cross your left leg over your right so your left ankle rests on your right thigh. Grasp your left knee with both hands and pull it toward the middle of your chest until you feel a gentle stretch in your glutes. Hold for 30 seconds, and then repeat on the other side. Repeat two more times on both legs. You can perform this stretch several times a day if your glutes are really tight.

PIGEON STRETCHES

This move is a little tricky. Face the floor on your hands and knees. Take your right leg and cross the lower part of that leg under your chest while straightening your left leg behind you. Support your upper body on your hands, or lower down to your elbows if you can. You will feel the stretch in your hip and butt. Hold for 10 to 15 seconds; then switch sides. Perform 3 sets.

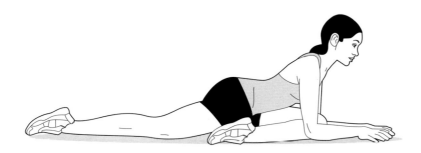

FOAM ROLLER EXERCISE

GLUTE ROLLS

Sit on your foam roller with your knees bent, feet flat on the floor. Cross your right leg over the front of your left thigh. Put your hands on the floor for support and roll your glutes back and forth from your hamstrings to your lower back for 30 seconds. Switch legs and repeat.

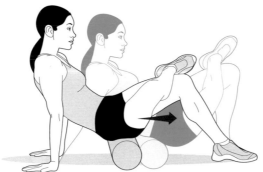

STRENGTH EXERCISES

MOUNTAIN CLIMBERS

You can do these on the floor or use a bench or step. Get into a pushup position with your arms straight, shoulders over your hands, and legs straight behind you and supported on your toes. Bring your right knee straight into your chest, and then extend it straight back to the starting position. Then bring your left knee into your chest and back. Alternate your legs and move as fast as you can. As you do these, you want to maintain good form; keep your back in a neutral position—not rounded, not drooping. The movement should come from your hips. Perform 15 reps, counting right and left together as 1 rep. Do 3 sets.

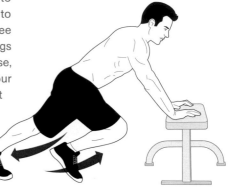

STEP INSIDE THE GYM WITH ME

To watch a video showing how to do plyometric jump squats, turn to page 200.

PLYOMETRIC JUMP SQUATS

Stand tall with your feet a little more than shoulder-width apart and toes turned slightly outward. Put your arms straight out in front of you. Squat down, pushing your butt back while keeping your upper body tall. (If you can get your butt down below your knees, this move will give your glutes a good workout.) Now explode up as high as you can and land softly. Maintain a good anatomical position and control your movement. Do 3 sets of 15.

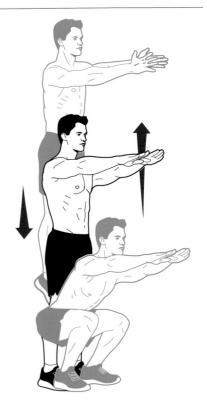

REVERSE LUNGES WITH REACH BACK

Stand tall with your arms straight down at your sides. Engage your core and lunge back with your right leg, lowering your body until your knee nearly touches the floor. As you lunge, reach your arms back over your shoulders and to the left. Return to the starting position and perform a total of 15 reps. Then switch sides. Do 3 sets of 15 lunges on each side.

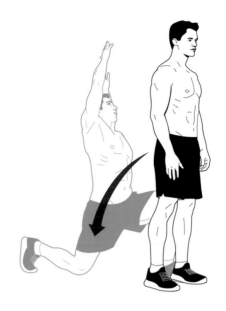

PLANKS

Get into a pushup position but bend your elbows and rest your weight on your forearms. Your body should form a straight line from your shoulders to your ankles. Engage your core, squeeze your glutes, and hold for 1 minute. Then roll to one side and hold your body up off the floor in a straight line from head to foot for 1 minute. Switch and do a plank on your other side.

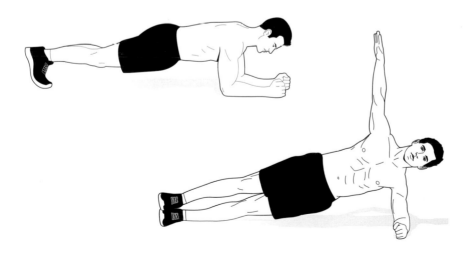

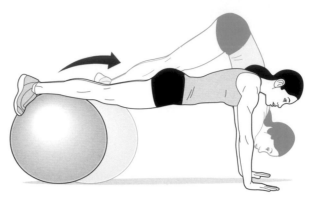

SWISS BALL PIKES

Rest your shins on top of a Swiss ball, and support your upper body with your hands flat on the floor and slightly more than shoulder-width apart, arms straight. Your body should form a straight line from your head to your ankles. Without bending your knees, roll the ball toward your chest by raising your hips as high as you can toward the ceiling. Pause, and then lower your hips as you roll the ball back to the starting position. Do 3 sets of 15 reps.

Note: If these are too difficult, begin with knee tucks, pulling the ball to your chest without raising your hips. Work your way up to the pike position as you get stronger and more stable.

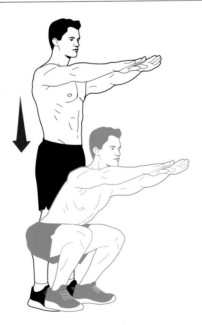

SQUATS

Stand tall with your feet shoulder-width apart. With your arms straight out in front of you, lower your body, bending your knees and pushing your butt back as if you are going to sit down in a chair until you reach a right angle at your knees. Pause, and then slowly push yourself back up to the starting position. Do 15 reps and up to 3 sets daily.

MULTIDIRECTIONAL LUNGES

Stand tall, keeping your trunk upright and stable, and lunge forward with your right leg as you lower your body until your back knee nearly touches the ground. Pause, and then push yourself back to the starting position. Then lunge forward with your left leg. Next, perform the same movement, lunging diagonally with both legs and on both sides. Finally, lunge back, alternating legs. Really use your core muscles to keep your upper body stable and upright as you do these. Repeat in all directions two more times for a total of 3 sets.

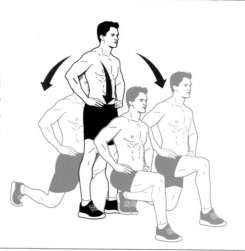

LOW SIDE-TO-SIDE LUNGES

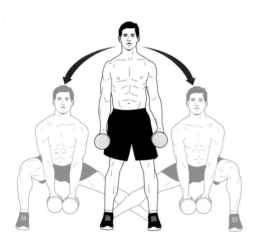

Stand with your feet shoulder-width apart and facing straight ahead. Clasp your hands in front of your chest (or use dumbbells as illustrated). Shift your weight to your right leg and lower your body, bending your right knee and pushing your butt back. Keep your left leg straight and left foot flat on the floor. Without raising yourself all the way to standing, shift the movement to the left. As you do this exercise, engage your core to keep your upper body vertical. Alternate back and forth for a total of 15 reps—right and left together is 1 rep. Perform 3 sets of 15.

Challenge move: You can add dumbbells to this exercise. Hold them straight down in front of you with your palms facing in as you shift from one leg to the other.

DIAGONAL LUNGES

Stand tall, keeping your trunk upright and stable, and lunge diagonally to your right with your right leg as you lower your body until your back knee nearly touches the ground. Pause, and then push yourself back to the starting position. Really use your core muscles to keep your upper body stable and upright; you don't want to bend forward or side to side. Complete 15 reps and switch sides, lunging with your left leg. Perform 3 sets of 15 reps on each side.

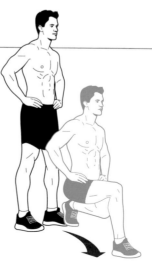

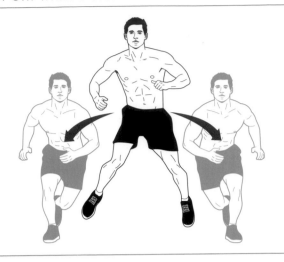

SKATERS

Stand with a slight forward bend and jump sideways from right to left. As you land on your left foot, bring your right foot back and behind your left leg and your right arm across the front of your body. Then jump from your left foot back to the right. That's 1 rep. Do 3 sets of 15 reps.

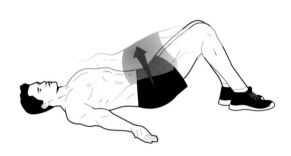

GLUTEAL BRIDGES

Lie on your back with your knees bent and feet flat on the floor. Place your arms straight down at your sides, palms up. Raise your hips until your knees, hips, and shoulders form a straight line. You should feel your glutes flex. Hold for several seconds, and then lower your body until it almost touches the floor. That's 1 rep. Repeat. Do 3 sets of 15.

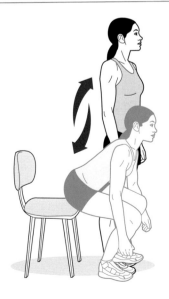

CHAIR SQUATS

Stand in front of a chair and do a squat onto the chair; stand back up and repeat. Gradually work your way up to 6 sets of 15 reps. Also, do single-leg squats onto the chair; again, gradually work your way up to 6 sets of 15 reps.

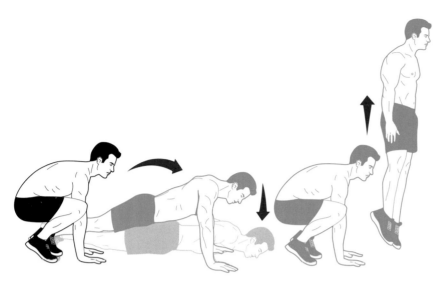

STEP INSIDE THE GYM WITH ME

To watch a video showing how to do burpees, turn to page 206.

BURPEES

Stand with your feet shoulder-width apart and arms at your sides. Lower into a deep squat, place your hands flat on the floor, and kick your legs straight back so you are in a pushup position. Do a pushup if you can, and then quickly bring your legs back to the squat position and stand up. That's 1 rep. Aim for as many as you can muster up to 3 sets of 15. You can make this exercise easier by supporting your upper body on a bench or step.

DUMBBELL SPLIT SQUATS

Hold a dumbbell in each hand, arms straight down at your sides. Place your feet in a staggered position, 2 to 3 feet apart. Slowly lower your body as far as you can and pause; then push yourself back up to the starting position as quickly as you can. Use your core muscles to keep your upper body vertical. Do 15 reps and switch sides. Aim for 3 sets of 15 reps on each side.

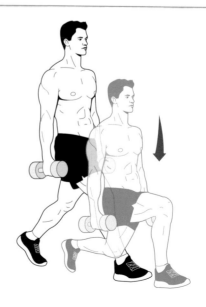

139

STANDING RESISTANCE-BAND HIP ABDUCTIONS

Secure a mini band to a sturdy object. Standing with your right leg next to the object, loop the band around your left ankle. Starting with your legs together, raise your left leg straight out to the side as far as you can. Pause, and then return to the starting position. Do 15 reps; then switch sides. Aim for 3 sets of 15 on each side.

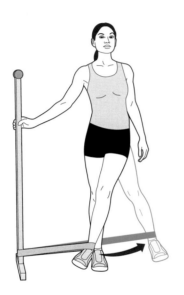

LATERAL BAND WALKS

Place a mini band around your legs just above your knees. Take small steps to your right for 20 feet, and then sidestep back to your left for 20 feet. As you do this exercise, keep your feet apart; don't bring them together. You want to maintain tension in the band. Repeat two more times in each direction.

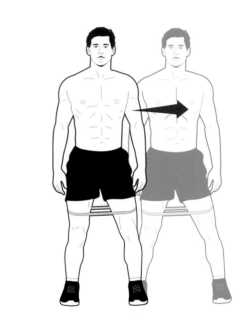

FIRE HYDRANT IN-OUTS

Get down on your hands and knees with your palms flat on the floor and shoulder-width apart. Pull your right knee in toward your chest and, keeping that knee bent, raise your thigh out to the side without moving your hips. Kick your raised leg straight back until it is in line with your torso. That's 1 rep. Repeat on your left side and alternate sides for a total of 15 reps. Aim for 3 sets of 15.

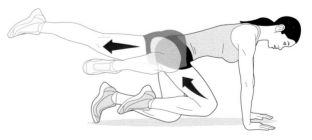

CHAPTER 9

YOUR LOWER BACK

You may not think your lower back has much of a role in running, but when you run, you hold your body vertical, of course, sometimes for a very long time.

Your core muscles support your spine and lower back, and your core, hips, glutes, and hamstrings together form one big stability machine, so weakness in any one of those muscles forces the others to take up the slack. If you have weak hip and gluteal muscles, for example, as they become fatigued during a run, your lower back is forced to work harder to keep you upright and stable, and you become vulnerable to injury.

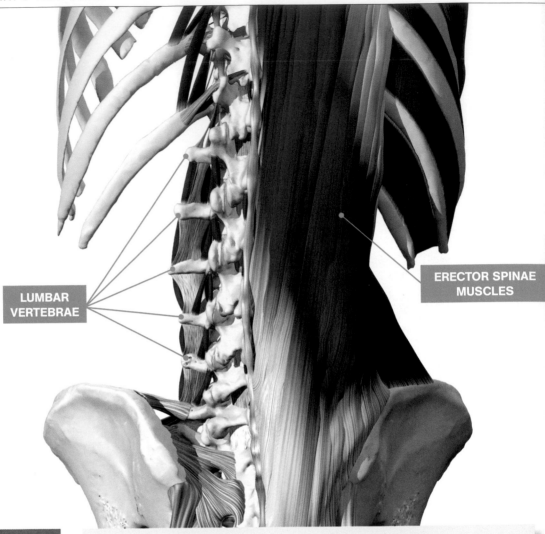

LUMBAR VERTEBRAE

ERECTOR SPINAE MUSCLES

STEP INTO MY OFFICE

Blipp this page to view a video about various sources of back pain and how to deal with it.

Where Does It Hurt?

1. Muscular pain that comes on suddenly in your lower back is indicative of a ***muscle spasm***. Your muscles will feel as though they have locked up, and the pain can be severe and debilitating. You will ***not*** feel the shooting pain characteristic of sciatic or discogenic pain.

2. Pain in your lower back that is associated with shooting pains down the back of one or both legs indicates ***sciatica*** or ***discogenic pain.*** A pinched nerve causes this discomfort, so you will not experience the muscle-gripping sensation that you would feel with a spasm.

3. If you feel a chronic general achiness across the whole area of your lower back, you may have ***arthritis.***

Lower-Back Spasm

Put too much strain on the muscles of your lower back and they will get angry.

SYMPTOMS

You will feel a sudden, gripping muscular pain across both sides of your spine, as if your muscles have locked up. The pain can be severe and debilitating.

WHAT'S GOING ON

The muscles in your back have spontaneously contracted. This most often happens with twisting, bending, pushing, and pulling motions, but it may occur during a long run if your muscles are weak or tight, or if you have a muscular imbalance that throws off your alignment or running mechanics and puts extra strain on your lower back.

The paraspinal muscles (aka erector spinae) run along both sides of your spine, from your hip to the base of your skull. They are among the strongest in your body, and they enable you to move, twist, and bend your spine. During running, they work to keep your upper body upright, and when weak or tight, they can go into spasm.

WHAT TO DO

(Instructions for the following stretches and exercises appear at the end of this chapter.)

- You will want to lie down and curl up into a ball until the pain goes away—but don't. Keep moving, even if it means shuffling around the house; movement helps relieve the spasm and prevents your muscles from losing their conditioning.

- Apply ice for 15 minutes four to six times a day for the first 2 days. After 48 hours, place a heating pad against your lower back for 15 minutes four to six times a day until you feel relief.

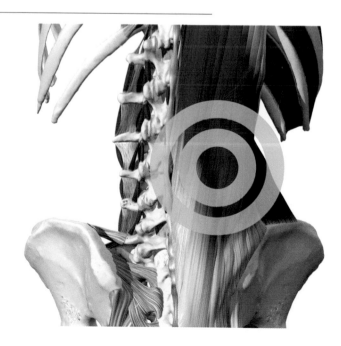

- Take an anti-inflammatory, such as ibuprofen or naproxen, to help with pain and any inflammation.

- During the acute phase of the spasm, don't stretch your lower-back muscles, but do loosen your muscles with the hamstring roll and lying glutes stretch. Tight hamstrings in particular will pull on your lower spine and accentuate its curvature.

- Try different therapies. There are several ways to treat back pain, and what works for one person may not work for another. Some of my patients respond well to massage therapy; others find that acupuncture helps; some may find relief from muscle pain with chiropractic. So if one treatment doesn't help, try another.

- If you are not getting relief from back pain or if the pain is severe, see your doctor. Muscular spasms don't require a doctor's care, but your physician can prescribe muscle relaxants if other treatments aren't working. Also, you will want to get checked out to see if there are any underlying issues, such as osteoarthritis, spinal stenosis, or a herniated disk. An x-ray will help diagnose any bone issues, and an MRI will help identify disk problems.

- When the pain subsides, you can start running again. You will also want to begin reconditioning your lower-back muscles as well as your core, glutes, and hamstrings. Do planks and hip raises, and use your foam roller on your hamstrings. Go slowly and increase reps and intensity as it becomes more comfortable. When you are completely free of pain, up your conditioning with the exercises recommended in "Prevention" below.

PREVENTION

To prevent back pain, you need to work on strength and flexibility all through your kinetic chain. Your spine and spinal muscles get lots of support from your core. In addition, tightness or weakness in your glutes, hips, quads, and hamstrings will impact the muscles in your lower back, putting more strain on those muscles and setting them up for a spasm.

- Do the IronStrength workout once or twice a week (see Chapter 12 and watch the videos).

- Use your foam roller every day (see page 210) to keep muscles flexible.

- Perform the Swiss ball pike, hip raise, reverse hip raise, back extensions, and cobra (shown at the end of this chapter) daily.

Discogenic Back Pain or Sciatica

The sciatic nerve—the source of this pain—is the largest nerve in your lower back and runs from your lumbar spine down both of your legs. Squeeze the nerve near its source and, like a little bolt of electricity, pain shoots down to your toes.

SYMPTOMS

You will feel pain in your lower back that worsens when you bend forward and shoots down the back of your leg. Often the pain will localize in the butt, confusing it with piriformis syndrome.

WHAT'S GOING ON

You have a pinched nerve in your spine. If you have a herniated or slipped disk, it means that a part of the lining of the disk has torn due to an impact, wrenching of your spine, or degeneration, and the material inside the disk is bulging out. When that bulging material presses against a nerve, it hurts. Sciatica refers specifically to impingement of the sciatic nerve.

WHAT TO DO

(Instructions for the following stretches and exercises appear at the end of this chapter.)

- Make an appointment with your doctor. You need to have an MRI to determine exactly what's going on in your spine. Once your physician has confirmed a diagnosis, he may recommend an injection of cortisone or an anesthetic to relieve the pain. In addition, your doctor may suggest physical therapy, which will help with the pain and condition your muscles to better support your spine. While the stretching and strengthening I recommend here will help, a physical therapist

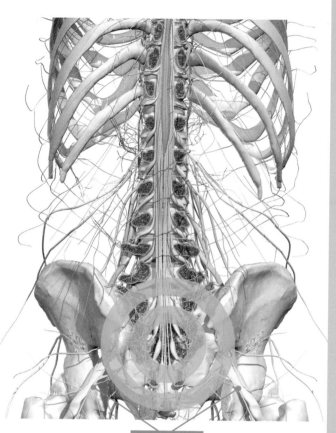

SCIATIC NERVE

will be able to direct treatment specific to your individual case and teach you proper form with the exercises he prescribes.

- Movement with lower-back injuries is a good thing. It can prevent spasms and keep your muscles from losing their conditioning. If you can run without pain affecting your form, great. If not, find something you can do, even if it's a slow shuffle around the house, to keep moving.

- Apply ice for 15 minutes four to six times a day for the first 2 days. After 48 hours, place a heating pad against your lower back for 15 minutes four to six times a day until you feel relief.

- Take an anti-inflammatory, such as ibuprofen or naproxen, to help relieve pain and inflammation.

- During the acute phase of the spasm, don't stretch your lower-back muscles but do loosen your glutes, hamstrings, and hip flexors with the hamstring roll and lying

glutes stretch. Tight hamstrings will pull on your lower spine and accentuate its curvature.

- There are several ways to treat back pain, and what works for one person may not work for another. Some of my patients respond well to massage therapy; others find that acupuncture helps; some may find relief from muscle pain with chiropractic. So if one treatment doesn't help you, try another.

- With home treatment, pain usually subsides in about 3 weeks and you can resume serious running again. You will also want to begin reconditioning your lower-back muscles as well as your core, glutes, and hamstrings. Do planks and hip raises, and use your foam roller on your hamstrings. Go slowly, and increase reps and intensity as it becomes more comfortable. When you are completely free of pain, up your conditioning with the exercises recommended below.

PREVENTION

The muscles in your legs, hips, core, and back work together. Focusing only on the muscles in your back does not solve back problems. Weak or tight hamstrings, quadriceps, glutes, hips, or core muscles all can give you back trouble because a deficiency in one part of the kinetic chain puts more pressure on another to work extra hard. And with a repetitive activity like running, that extra work results in injury.

- Do the IronStrength workout once or twice a week (see Chapter 12 and watch the videos) to build total-body strength.

- Use your foam roller (see page 210) every day.

- Perform planks, back extensions, the Swiss ball pike, the hip raise, the reverse hip raise, and the cobra (all shown at the end of this chapter) daily.

Arthritis of the Spine

Unfortunately, there is no cure for arthritis. It will get worse over time, but I promise that you can ease the pain, slow down the progression, and keep running.

SYMPTOMS

You will feel chronic achiness across your lower back with no associated shooting pains.

WHAT'S GOING ON

Osteoarthritis is the wearing out of the tissue between the bones of a joint, leaving bone to grind on bone. It commonly affects runners in their sixties or seventies. Former injuries increase your risk of arthritis. Genetics, overuse, and poor biomechanics also may play a role.

WHAT TO DO

- If you think you have arthritis, see your doctor, who will order an x-ray to confirm a diagnosis. He should also do a full assessment of your strength, flexibility, and foot mechanics in addition to reviewing your running shoes, where you run, and your training.

- Keep moving. Research shows that regular activity is better than rest for keeping arthritic joints lubricated and for slowing wear and tear. But cut back on your mileage, using pain as your guide. If you become hungry for more cardio, consider nonimpact activities, such as cycling, the elliptical trainer, ElliptiGO, swimming, or pool running.

- Take an anti-inflammatory, such as ibuprofen or naproxen, to help relieve pain.

- Strengthen your core, glutes, and hamstrings by doing planks, back extensions, the Swiss ball pike, the hip raise, the reverse hip raise, and the cobra (all shown at the end of this chapter) daily.

- Check your stride length and cadence. Count every time your right foot hits the ground, and aim for 85 to 90 footstrikes a minute. With a shorter stride, your foot hits the ground closer to the center of your body mass, which eases the impact of running.

- Take your running to softer surfaces. Asphalt is softer than concrete, but grass and dirt or cinder trails are better still.

PREVENTION

Build strength and flexibility in your kinetic chain. Strong muscles in your core, glutes, hips, hamstrings, and quads will take some of the load off your back, which reduces pain and will slow the progression of arthritis.

- Do the IronStrength workout once or twice a week (see Chapter 12 and watch the videos).

- To keep your muscles flexible—tight muscles put more pressure on your spine—use your foam roller daily (see page 210).

FOAM ROLLER EXERCISES

HAMSTRING ROLLS

Position your foam roller under your leg just above your right knee and straighten your leg. Cross your left leg over your right at the ankle. Place your hands on the floor for support and roll your leg back and forth from your knee to your butt for 30 seconds, then switch legs. If this is too painful, uncross your legs and roll one at a time, or if you have a long roller, roll both legs at the same time.

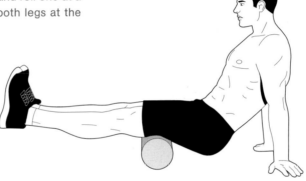

STRETCHES

LYING GLUTES STRETCHES

Lie on your back on the floor and bend your hips and knees so your calves are parallel to the floor. Cross your left leg over your right so your left ankle rests on your right thigh. Grasp your left knee with both hands and pull it toward the middle of your chest until you feel a gentle stretch in your glutes. Hold for 30 seconds, then repeat on the other side. Repeat two more times on both legs. You can perform this stretch several times a day if your glutes are really tight.

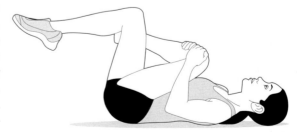

STRENGTH EXERCISES

PLANKS

Get into a pushup position but bend your elbows and rest your weight on your forearms. Your body should form a straight line from your shoulders to your ankles. Engage your core, squeeze your glutes, and hold for 1 minute. Then roll to one side and hold your body up off the floor in a straight line from head to foot for 1 minute. Switch and do a plank on your other side.

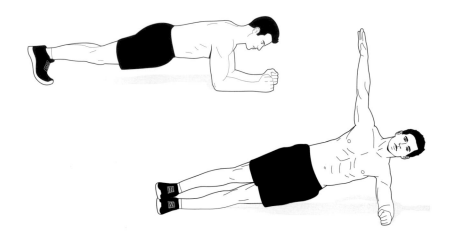

BACK EXTENSIONS

Position yourself in the back extension station and hook your feet under the leg anchors. Keeping your back naturally arched, place your hands behind your head and lower your upper body as far as you comfortably can. Squeeze your glutes and raise your torso until it's in line with your lower body. Pause, then slowly lower your torso to the starting position.

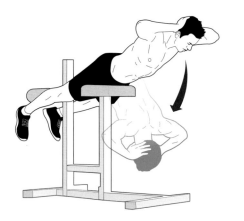

SWISS BALL PIKES

Rest your shins on top of a Swiss ball and support your upper body with your hands flat on the floor and slightly more than shoulder-width apart, arms straight. Your body should form a straight line from your head to your ankles. Without bending your knees, roll the ball toward your chest by raising your hips as high as you can toward the ceiling. Pause, and then lower your hips as you roll the ball back to the starting position. Do 3 sets of 15 reps.

Note: If these are too difficult, begin with knee tucks, pulling the ball in to your chest without raising your hips. Work your way up to the pike position as you get stronger and more stable.

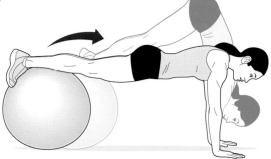

REVERSE HIP RAISES

Lie facedown on a bench with your torso on the bench and your hips off it. Keeping your legs nearly straight, lift them until they are in line with your torso. Squeeze your glutes, raise your hips, and pause; lower to the starting position. Do 3 sets of 15.

Note: You can also do this exercise with a Swiss ball, placing your hands flat on the floor in front of you for support.

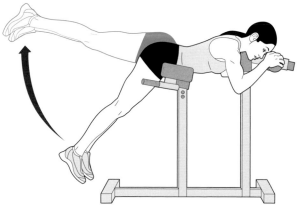

HIP RAISES

Lie on your back on the floor with your knees bent and feet flat on the floor. Squeezing your glutes, raise your hips until your body forms a straight line from your shoulders to your knees. Pause for 5 seconds, and then lower to the starting position. Do 3 sets of 15.

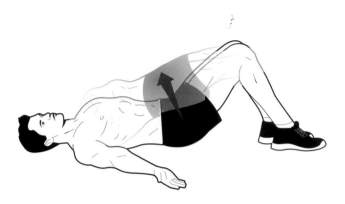

COBRA

Lie facedown on the floor with your legs straight behind you and your arms straight down next to your sides, palms down. Contract your glutes and lower-back muscles as you raise your head, chest, arms, and legs off the floor and rotate your arms so your thumbs point toward the ceiling. Hold for 30 seconds, and then relax back to the floor for 5 seconds. Repeat three times.

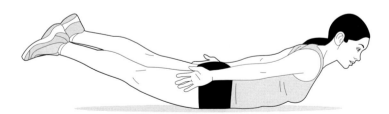

CHAPTER 10
YOUR UPPER BODY

Most of the work of running takes place below the waist. You're not going to strain your abs or your pectoral muscles on your daily 5-miler. But runners do experience chest pain; it could be as harmless as side stitches or as serious as heart-related pain. Either way, you will want to be prepared to handle it.

Finally, we reach the top of your body—command central, where all movement originates. Yes, running can even cause pain in your head. But what exactly is it that hurts when you have a headache? Not your brain; there's no sensation in brain tissue. Pain can come from the nerves of your scalp, the blood vessels on the surface of your brain, or the muscles in your head.

Angina Pectoris (aka Chest Pain)

Chest pain strikes fear in the hearts of just about everybody. And for good reason: Heart disease is the number-one killer of men and women. And if I'm going to be honest with you—which I am—there is a tiny increase in risk of heart attack during any intense physical activity. A tiny one. The American College of Sports Medicine estimates that the chance of a cardiac patient having a heart attack during strenuous physical activity is 1 in 100,000 to 300,000 hours of exercise. So that means if you run 10 hours a week, you would need to run 10,000 weeks to log 100,000 hours. And 10,000 weeks is 192 years.

Take into account also that people who regularly do some sort of cardiovascular exercise have a stronger heart, lower blood pressure, and lower cholesterol, and you can see that running is one of the best things you can do for your heart.

It is possible to have chest pain that is unrelated to angina. *Costochondritis* is an irritation of the sternum where the ribs attach. Regardless, any chest pain, as well as shortness of breath, needs to be checked out by your doctor.

SYMPTOMS

- Pain, squeezing, or pressure in the center of the chest

- Possible discomfort in your neck, jaw, shoulder, back, or arm

- Possible shortness of breath, nausea, vomiting, or mid- to lower-back pain for women

- Symptoms last about 5 minutes or less and go away when you stop running

WHAT'S GOING ON

Angina pectoris occurs when your heart doesn't get as much blood and oxygen as it needs. Plaque (a fatty buildup) on the walls of your coronary arteries narrows the passage that blood flows through. When you're running and your heart is working hard, it needs more oxygen. If not enough blood is flowing through the coronary arteries to meet those needs, you will experience chest pain or angina. In addition to physical exertion, emotional stress and very hot or very cold temperatures can trigger angina.

If you have heart disease and regularly experience angina, you are familiar with what triggers it and what it feels like. If it begins to occur more easily—possibly even at rest—and more frequently, you may have unstable

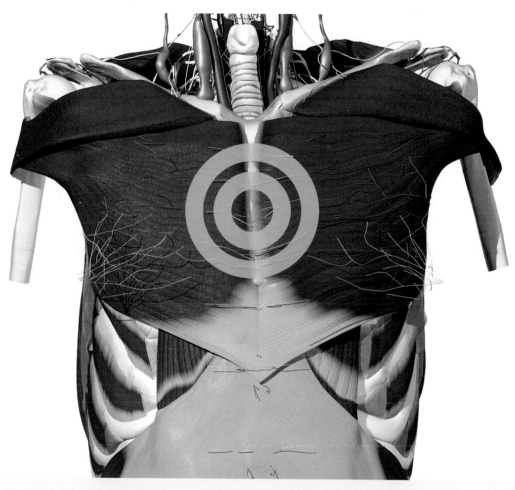

Where Does It Hurt?

1. Pain, squeezing, and pressure in the center of your chest are classic signs of *angina.* These symptoms may be accompanied by pain in your neck, jaw, shoulder, or arm.

2. Shortness of breath, wheezing, and tightness in the chest are all symptoms of *exercise-induced bronchospasm.*

3. Sudden, intense throbbing usually on both sides of your head indicates an *exercise-induced headache.*

4. Though we tend to think of *migraine headaches* as excruciating, the pain can be mild to agonizing. Migraines occur on only one side of your head and in many cases are accompanied by auras (visual disturbances), nausea, tingling, or other nervous system disorders.

angina, which means the plaque in one or more of your coronary arteries has ruptured, and you are at risk for heart attack. *Get to the ER.*

WHAT TO DO

- If you experience the symptoms described here, stop running and get to the emergency room, where an EKG and blood tests will be performed to determine if you have had a heart attack. A follow-up with a cardiologist may include a stress test with imaging to further see what's going on with your arteries. Depending on the amount of blockage, treatment might be as simple as a prescription for nitroglycerin or as complex as surgery.

- If you have been diagnosed with stable angina, your doctor will likely have prescribed nitroglycerin, which relaxes blood vessels and increases bloodflow to the heart. When an episode of angina occurs during a run, stop and take a nitroglycerin pill. And it's quits until you are cleared by your doc! Don't mess with chest pain, my friends.

PREVENTION

- Keep running. Though it can't alter your genetics or erase damage from prior health issues, such as smoking and obesity, running strengthens your heart muscles, builds more blood vessels around the heart, and lowers the key contributors to heart disease: blood pressure, cholesterol, and triglycerides (fatty acids) in the blood. I must stress here that if you have been diagnosed with heart disease, your running plan and intensity need to be cleared with your cardiologist before you run!

- Take low-dose aspirin every day if recommended by your doctor, which "thins" the blood to help prevent clots from forming and reduces your risk of a cardiac event.

- Follow a diet low in saturated fat, high in fiber, and that includes monounsaturated fats, such as olive oil (see Chapter 15 for details about a healthy diet for runners).

Exercise-Induced Bronchospasm (aka Exercise-Induced Asthma)

Exercise-induced bronchospasm (EIB) used to be called and is still often referred to as exercise-induced asthma, but asthma is a chronic condition unrelated to exercise. A bronchospasm is a tightening and narrowing of the air passages that lead to your lungs. Though individuals who suffer from asthma are at great risk for EIB, you don't have to be an asthmatic to experience it. If a bronchospasm occurs on a run, stop. But don't be concerned that you will have to stop running for life, because you won't. With the right strategies in place, you can have a long and happy running life.

SYMPTOMS

- Shortness of breath, wheezing, tightness in the chest, and coughing indicate EIB. Generally, you begin to experience symptoms anywhere from 5 to 15 minutes into your run, and symptoms continue after you have stopped.
- EIB usually occurs when you are running in cold, dry conditions.

WHAT'S GOING ON

When you breathe, air is warmed and moistened as it moves through your nose and along your airways. But when the air you're breathing is particularly cold and dry and most of it is bypassing your nose and entering through your mouth, coming and going in quick breaths as you inhale and exhale rapidly during running, the cold air doesn't get warmed. It hits the lining of your airways, irritates the tissue, and triggers the tightening of muscle and narrowing of the passages. Some runners also find that pollen and pollution trigger an attack.

WHAT TO DO

See your physician for a thorough exam, which may include an exercise test designed to elicit a bronchospasm. If a diagnosis is confirmed, your doctor may prescribe medication: a bronchodilator or an anti-inflammatory. A bronchodilator helps relax your airway to keep it open. It's administered with an inhaler and can be used before or during a run. Anti-inflammatories such as inhaled corticosteroids reduce the sensitivity of your air passages and are used prior to running. One or both of these medications should give you relief.

PREVENTION

- When temperatures drop, wear a face mask or cover your mouth with a scarf to warm and moisten air as you inhale. (Just don't jog into your neighborhood bank.)

- Consider running on the treadmill on days that are especially cold or when pollen or pollution is high.

- Avoid doing speedwork outdoors on frigid days since intense running requires rapid breaths and increases your risk of EIB.

- Take advantage of the EIB refractory period—a time period of up to 2 hours immediately following a bronchospasm during which your body is less likely to react to triggers. If you have an intense run planned, warm up 45 minutes to an hour ahead of time, rest, and then run.

Exercise-Induced Headache

I like to describe this as when the runner's high turns into the runner's headache.

SYMPTOMS

Exercise-induced headaches fall into two categories: primary and secondary. The primary kind is characterized by sudden, intense throbbing usually on both sides of your head during or after a run. It may last anywhere from 5 minutes to 2 days.

The more severe secondary headache also produces sudden, intense throbbing pain but may also cause dizziness, vomiting, blurred vision, or neck rigidity. It may last a day to several days. *If you experience these symptoms, go to the emergency room.*

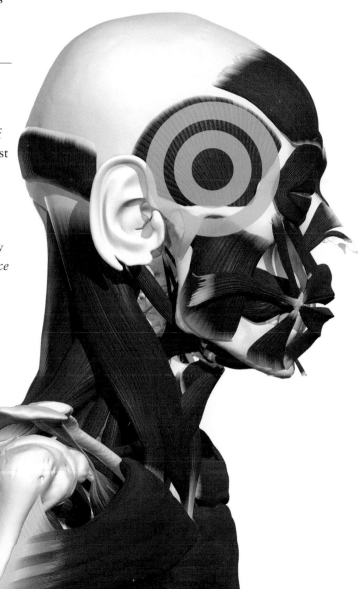

WHAT'S GOING ON

No one knows what causes a primary exercise-induced headache, but experts theorize that the dilation of the blood vessels in your brain, which occurs during running, may be the trigger. Exercising in hot weather or at a high altitude or having a family history of migraines may make you more susceptible to these headaches.

Secondary exercise-induced headaches have an underlying cause, which could be as simple as a sinus infection or as serious as bleeding between the brain and the membrane that surrounds it, abnormalities in some of the blood vessels of the brain, or even a tumor. I repeat: If you experience the symptoms of a secondary exercise-induced headache, go to the ER.

WHAT TO DO

- At the first sign of pain, drink a couple cups of water, which studies have shown may alleviate the headache within 30 minutes.

- Take acetaminophen or ibuprofen.

- Try placing a cold cloth on your forehead or the back of your neck for 10 to 15 minutes. If your blood vessels are dilated, the cold may constrict them and provide relief.

- Try acupressure with these two methods: (1) Pinch the webbed area between your forefinger and thumb and apply pressure in a circular motion; then do the same on the other hand. (2) Use your thumbs to apply circular pressure at the back of your head just beneath your skull and midway between the bony bumps behind your ears and the middle of your skull.

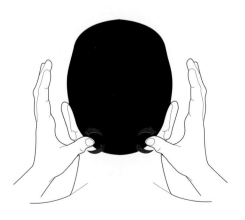

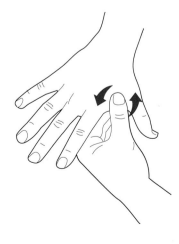

- Try this: Place a pencil between your teeth but don't bite down. This relaxes your jaw muscles.

- The first time you experience a sudden and intense headache during or after a run, see your doctor, even if the pain lasts only a few minutes. It is likely that nothing serious is going on, but it's best to find that out from your doctor.

- If you have symptoms of a secondary exercise-induced headache, go to the ER. The doctor will order a CT scan or an MRI to see what's going on inside your head, and she may prescribe a prescription anti-inflammatory or blood pressure medication.

PREVENTION

- If you tend to get exercise-induced headaches when running in heat and humidity, plan your runs for the early morning—the coolest time of day—or seek out a treadmill in an air-conditioned location. If neither of these options works for you, try taking your preferred pain reliever an hour before you run.

- If high altitudes are your nemesis, taking pain meds an hour before you run may prevent a headache.

- Always do a warmup before a speed workout or a race, when the intensity of your running might trigger a headache.

Migraine

The dreaded migraine. For many people, the side effects are worse than the headache.

SYMPTOMS

- You will have a mild to severe headache on one side of your head, which may be accompanied by nausea and vomiting as well as sensitivity to light and noise.

- The migraine may be preceded by auras—nervous system disturbances usually related to vision, including blind spots, flashes of light, and seeing shapes or patterns.

- You may have tingling in an arm or a leg or have trouble speaking.

- If you get migraines regularly, you may discover that a day or two prior to an attack you suffer from diarrhea, constipation, a stiff neck, irritability, depression, hyperactivity, or food cravings.

WHAT'S GOING ON

Unfortunately, we don't really know exactly how or why migraines happen. Changes in the brain stem or imbalances in brain chemicals, including serotonin, may play a role. Serotonin helps to regulate levels of pain in the nervous system, and levels drop during a migraine; this triggers the production of other brain chemicals called neuropeptides that travel to the outer layer of the brain and may cause pain.

What *do* we know? That the predisposition for migraines is genetic and that there are several environmental triggers: hormonal shifts, foods, alcohol, bright lights, stress, dehydration, certain smells, weather, and lack of sleep. We also know that migraines are three times more common in women than in men.

WHAT TO DO

- If you feel a migraine coming on during a run, stop and walk back home. Exercise during a migraine dilates blood vessels, and dilated blood vessels may play a role in headache pain.

- As soon as you feel a migraine coming on, take whatever over-the-counter or prescription medication brings you relief: aspirin, anti-inflammatories (such as ibuprofen or naproxen), acetaminophen, or medications sold specifically for migraine relief, which combine the usual headache relievers with caffeine.

- Drink a few cups of water, since dehydration makes headaches worse and may have caused your migraine.

- Researchers have long believed dilation of the blood vessels in the brain is at the root of migraine pain, so try drinking a cup of caffeinated coffee. The caffeine will constrict blood vessels. Bonus: It boosts the effect of pain meds.

- After using the aforementioned treatments, many migraine sufferers find that the best course of action is to lie down in a dark room until the migraine passes.

- Write down in a journal all possible triggers that occurred around your attack: what you ate and drank, the weather, your stress level, whether your eyes were exposed to bright lights; women, take note of where you are in your menstrual cycle. Keeping a journal will help you pinpoint your triggers, and if you see a physician to discuss your migraines, you will have a record of the possible environmental triggers.

- Some people get relief with alternative methods: acupuncture, biofeedback, the herbs feverfew and butterbur, vitamin B_2 (riboflavin), magnesium, and coenzyme Q10.

- If your migraines are mild enough that you can get through them with the remedies described here, you don't need to see a doctor. But if your headaches are severe, make an appointment to get an exam and discuss treatment options. Several prescription medications are effective at preventing and relieving pain: triptans, ergots, even Botox injections. In addition, some cardiovascular meds as well as certain antidepressants have a preventive effect.

PREVENTION

- Drink plenty of fluids daily. Dehydration may trigger migraines.

- Alcohol is at the top of the list of the most common food triggers of migraines. Among these offending beverages, red wine is the culprit more often than white; beer, champagne, and eggnog are frequently reported to cause migraines; and dark-colored spirits, such as scotch, rye, and bourbon, appear to be more evil than white spirits, such as gin and vodka.

- Get enough sleep: Strive for 7 to 8 hours a night.

- Stay committed to making notes in a headache journal every time you have a migraine, and refer to that journal to search for a pattern. Once you have identified your triggers, you can avoid them, and the headaches.

CHAPTER 11

Blisters, Bonking, and Other Annoying Maladies

There are big injuries—stress fractures, plantar fasciitis, runner's knee—that can sideline you for weeks, even months. Then there's the small stuff, like blisters, bunions, and chafing.

These minor maladies won't derail your training, but some of them can prevent you from grabbing that PR in your next race, a few can blow up into big problems if you aren't careful, and all of them are really annoying. Let's take a look at how to treat blisters and a bunch of other bothersome afflictions common among runners, and I will tell you how to prevent them so they never bother you again.

ABRASIONS

I know—you're thinking, "Abrasions? Running? Really?" Think trails; they're a minefield of rocks, roots, and ruts just waiting to take you down. The road? Especially postwinter—prime pothole season—maybe a little uneven pavement trips you up. And we have all witnessed some of the world's best tangle on the track. Lose your footing; slide across some granite, asphalt, tartan; and you will leave some skin behind.

What to Do

1. Gently scrub the abrasion using a clean cloth with mild soap and water to remove any dirt. It's going to sting, but you're tough. If you see any big pieces of debris, use tweezers to remove them.

2. Apply a triple-antibiotic ointment, like Neosporin, over the entire area, and a layer of petroleum jelly on top of that (which will prevent the bandage you're going to apply next from sticking to your raw flesh); then cover the area with a sterile gauze pad and use tape to secure it to your skin.

3. Take an anti-inflammatory such as ibuprofen or naproxen to relieve the throbbing.

4. Change the dressing once a day. The abrasion may ooze and be gooey, which is normal. Big abrasions usually heal from the deeper layers of the skin upward and from the edges toward the center.

Prevention

There may be nothing that will stop you from falling if you stumble over a tree root on a trail or your toe catches a big crack in the pavement, but with the right strength training you can improve your stability and balance and significantly bump up your chances of staying upright when the path tries to topple you.

- Do the IronStrength workout once or twice a week (see Chapter 12 and watch the videos).

- Trail running might be your nemesis, but it teaches your muscles how to perform on uneven surfaces so you become better at staying vertical.

ALLERGIES

Sniffling, sneezing, itchy eyes? All are symptoms of rhinitis or an allergy to pollen or other airborne irritants. If your allergies flare up during a run, let's hope you have a stash of tissues in your shorts pocket.

Prevention

Avoiding the enemy may not sound like the most courageous course of action, but it's the smartest when it comes to fighting allergies.

- Pollen counts are highest between 5 a.m. and 10 a.m., so plan your runs for late afternoon or evening if you can, and choose routes that steer clear of tall meadows, flower beds, and pollinating trees. This is not the time to go frolicking through the fields.

- Pollutants also trigger allergic reactions, so don't run on highly trafficked roads, and don't run during rush hour if you live along a busy commuter route.

- Wear sports sunglasses to keep irritants out of your eyes and a hat to prevent pollen from sticking to your hair.

- When you get home, toss your running gear in the laundry and take a shower to wash away any pollen that is clinging to your skin so it doesn't get up into your nose and become a nuisance as you carry it around with you for the rest of the day.

- You can check pollen counts in your area at the Web site of the American Academy of Allergy, Asthma & Immunology's National Allergy Bureau. On days when pollen is proliferating, you might want to consider taking your run to the treadmill.

THE BUZZ ON BEE STINGS

I would take a needle in the arm any day over the stinger of a wasp. And if you're someone who is highly allergic, you definitely don't want to meet up with these nasty arthropods on your run. Take the following precautions to sidestep the little buggers.

- Make yourself inconspicuous and choose neutrals over bright-colored clothing if you are allergic to bees.

- Run fragrance-free—no colognes, perfumes, or heavily scented lotions. Your natural scent is awesome; just make sure to shower, please.

- Avoid running near flower beds where bees and wasps like to hang out.

- If you have a severe allergy (i.e., you experience an anaphylactic reaction, which may include difficulty breathing; swelling in the face, mouth, or throat; hives; dizziness; rapid heartbeat), wear a medical ID bracelet and carry an EpiPen in case of an emergency.

- Keep in mind that warm, dry, breezy weather provides perfect conditions for allergens to take flight in abundance and travel through the air; consider running indoors on these days as well.

- If rhinitis regularly interferes with your running, talk with your pharmacist about taking an over-the-counter antihistamine—one that won't cause fatigue—before you run to prevent symptoms.

ANEMIA

Sometimes a female patient will tell me she feels tired all the time and lethargic when she runs, and she has no idea why. She gets plenty of sleep; she eats well. So I ask her about her training: Is she training hard? Putting in a lot of miles? And about her menstrual cycles—does she have heavy periods? If she answers yes to these questions, I'm thinking she has iron-deficiency anemia, and I recommend a blood test.

Your body uses iron to make red blood cells. If you are lacking iron, there aren't enough boxcars (red blood cells) to carry the precious cargo (oxygen) to the muscles and tissues that need them to function optimally. The result: Runners, and most often female runners due to the monthly loss of iron from menstruation, fatigue easily and feel like they are always "out of shape," even when they are well trained. In addition to fatigue and weakness, you may be pale under your fingernails and in the rims lining your eyelids, and you may have a rapid pulse, since your heart needs to work harder to move blood and oxygen around your body. Female runners don't just lose iron during menstruation either; when they run (and this goes for men too), they crush red blood cells with each footstrike. So if you love long distances, you destroy a lot of red blood cells. Then, if your diet is deficient in iron-rich foods—meat being one of the richest—you are looking at the trifecta of anemia risks.

What to Do

1. If you suspect that you may be anemic, see your doctor, who will order a blood test. If the results come back positive for an iron deficiency, your doc will discuss supplementation and dietary guidelines to raise your iron levels.

2. Even before you get your physician's dietary recommendations, you can add more iron-rich foods to your diet (see "Prevention").

3. Talk to your doc about checking in with a sports nutritionist who can help structure a diet with more iron included. If possible, find a nutritionist who runs so he will speak your language.

Prevention

Women need 15 milligrams of iron daily, but don't pop an iron supplement without first consulting your doctor; too much iron can damage your organs.

- Eat steak. Iron is most easily absorbed from animal proteins. But seriously, go for lean red meat, poultry, pork, and eggs.

- Are you a vegetarian or only an occasional carnivore? I have three words for you—beans and greens. Remember Popeye and his cans of spinach? Unfortunately, getting the iron you need from vegetarian sources isn't quite as easy as Popeye makes it seem. Your body has a tougher time absorbing iron from plant foods than from meat, but here's a tip: Vitamin C boosts iron absorption, so sprinkle a little lemon over your veggies, throw some bell peppers into your recipe, or enjoy a glass of OJ with your meal.

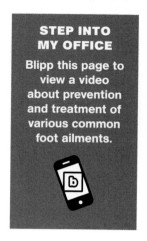

STEP INTO MY OFFICE

Blipp this page to view a video about prevention and treatment of various common foot ailments.

ATHLETE'S FOOT

It will set your foot on fire. The dreaded fungus tinea pedis makes camp in the warm, moist, cozy spaces between your toes. From there it spreads out to the rest of your foot and wreaks havoc, causing intense itching; burning; a scaly red rash; and possible swelling, cracking, even blisters.

Athlete's foot is very contagious, and you can easily pick it up in a locker room or bathroom or at the pool. Once on your foot and inside your sweaty running shoes, it thrives. Treat it immediately and thoroughly. A nasty case can take weeks to cure, and it will come back if you don't banish it. Now, get ready to take back your foot.

What to Do

1. Get relief by applying cool compresses to the infected area. Here's how: Dissolve one packet of Dome-boro powder or 2 tablespoons of Burow's solution (both available over-the-counter at pharmacies) in 1 pint of cold water. Soak a washcloth in the liquid; press the cloth into your sore, itchy skin; and hold it there for 15 to 20 minutes. Do this three or four times a day.

2. Purchase an over-the-counter antifungal medication. Choose a gel over a cream or lotion because the gels contain drying agents. Apply the gel to the infected area two or three times a day up until 2 weeks after the infection has cleared up.

3. When the acute phase of the attack has died down, remove any dead skin, which may house living fungi that can reinfect your foot. In the shower, scrub your entire foot lightly with a bristle brush.

Prevention

If you have never had athlete's foot, you will never want to get it, and if you have had it, you will never want to get it again. Here's how to keep tinea off your feet.

- This fungus easily finds its way from foot to foot, so wear shower shoes or flip-flops in public locker rooms and around pools—anywhere damp and where people go barefoot.

- After showering, allow your feet to dry for 5 to 10 minutes before putting on shoes. If you can't wait that long, use a hair dryer, wiggling your toes to dry between them.

- Have two pairs of running shoes and switch between them daily. It takes about 24 hours for athletic shoes to dry out after wearing them.

- Spray or dust the inside of your shoes with antifungal powder. You can also spray a cloth with a disinfectant like Lysol and wipe the insides of your shoes whenever you take them off.

BLACK TOENAILS

Black toenails are a rite of passage for many runners. Marathoners and runners who do a lot of downhills in shoes that don't have any room to spare keep banging their toes into the end or top of their shoes, and that repeated impact causes bruising or bleeding under the nail. Black toenails are really ugly, but generally they don't hurt and won't interfere with your training.

What to Do

Nothing. Eventually the toenail will come off as a new one grows in behind it. But you will never have to look at another black toenail again if you simply keep your toes from smashing against the top of your shoes.

Prevention

The long-term solution for most runners is to buy bigger running shoes. There should be a thumb's width of space between the end of your longest toe and the top of your shoe. You may need to go up a half to a full size from your street shoes. Here are a few more preventive tips.

- Trim your toenails regularly.

- Wear synthetic moisture-wicking socks to prevent things from getting slippery inside your shoes.

- Make sure your running shoes fit snugly at the heels and lace them to prevent your feet from sliding forward, especially for long runs and roads with lots of hills.

PS—I must also mention here that if you are looking to attract a mate who doesn't run, make sure you don't take off your socks until well into the courtship phase. Black toenails are normal for runners, but for the general public, not so much!

BLISTERS

Maybe you bought a new pair of running shoes and didn't break them in, or perhaps it rained on race day and your wet socks rubbed your skin relentlessly. Now you have blisters, one of the most annoying of annoying maladies.

Blisters pop up when repeated friction ruptures cells under the top layer of skin and plasma is released, forming a bubble.

What to Do

To pop or not to pop? That's the question runners ask me all the time. My rule is to leave a blister alone. Once you pop it, you have given bacteria an opening to get in there and cause an infection.

1. Cut a piece of moleskin in a doughnut shape, and place it over your blister so the blister is positioned in the open center of the moleskin. This should help reduce friction on the blister as it heals.

2. Now, if the blister is large and painful and hurts when you run on it, you have my permission to pop it. Using a needle sterilized in alcohol, poke a hole in the skin; let the fluid drain but keep the skin in place. Then wash the blister, apply an antibiotic ointment, and cover it with an adhesive bandage.

3. At night, remove the dressing, soak your foot in water for 10 minutes, and then let it air out for the rest of the night. Apply a fresh bandage in the morning.

4. If your blister itches or burns, apply a little Preparation H hemorrhoid cream. Weird, right? But it works.

5. If your blister starts to ooze pus and redden around the edges, you may have an infection. See your doctor immediately.

Prevention

- Make sure your running shoes fit well—snug but not tight—and your heel doesn't slip up and down at the back of the shoe.

- Don't take a brand-new pair of running shoes out for a 20-mile run, especially if you are trying out a new model. Break them in on shorter runs.

- Try double-layer socks. Blister-prone runners swear by them.

- Whatever type of sock you like, definitely choose those made with synthetic, breathable material so they won't become waterlogged if you happen to be running in the rain or sweat-logged in the heat.

- Try applying petroleum jelly to the areas of your feet prone to getting blisters.

STEP INTO MY OFFICE

Blipp this page to view a video addressing common questions patients often ask Dr. Metzl, including prevention and treatment of blisters.

BONKING

HYPOGLYCEMIA, AKA LOW BLOOD SUGAR

It's the fate of runners who run too far on too little fuel. Your body and your brain need glucose (blood sugar) to function. Once you use up what's in your bloodstream, your liver breaks down stored glycogen and releases more. And when you have burned through that, you are running on empty (pun intended). You feel weak, dizzy, and confused.

What to Do

Reach for the nearest and fastest injection of glucose—sports drinks or gels. If you happen to be running a marathon that offers orange sections at its water stops, grab them; orange juice delivers a fast shot of sugar into your bloodstream.

Prevention

You can prevent bonking by consuming plenty of carbs before a long run or marathon and carrying some with you (see Chapter 15 for more info about carbo-loading).

- Make sure your last meal before your long run or race is loaded with carbohydrates. (There's a strategy behind those prerace spaghetti dinners.)

- Eat an easily digested high-carb snack 30 minutes to an hour, depending on what your digestive system can handle, before you run—energy bars, bananas, cereal, something not too high in fiber, fat, or protein, which will slow digestion.

- Carry carbs in the form of sports gels in case you feel a little weak and woozy on the run.

HYPONATREMIA, AKA LOW BLOOD SODIUM

At mile 14 of the run stage in my first Ironman in Lake Placid, New York, a weird feeling came over me. I started losing awareness of where I was. I didn't seem to care about how I was doing in the race. In fact, I didn't care about much of anything. I'd had hypoglycemia before, but this was different. By mile 15, I just wanted to lie down at the side of the road and take a nap. Just at that point, I saw an old man holding a large jar of salt. I didn't know why, but I felt compelled to go to him. I opened my hand, took an entire handful of salt, and devoured it right in front of him. Almost immediately I felt better. My mind cleared; the world came into focus. On the way back, I passed my friend again and took another hit of salt. I smiled all the way to the finish. Without that salt, I would not have even reached the finish line.

Afterward, I thought more about what happened. As a doctor, I was fascinated by both the symptoms and the rapid cure. I did some research and soon learned that I had suffered a classic case of hyponatremia, a loss of sodium from the blood.

How do people end up with too little sodium in their bodies? Long, sweaty distance, that's how. Hyponatremia usually occurs during endurance events lasting more than 4 hours and in hot, humid conditions that cause you to sweat a lot. When you perspire, you lose fluids and electrolytes, such as sodium and potassium. How much you lose depends on the heat and humidity in the environment, on your genetics, and on your fitness level—the fitter you are, the more sweat you lose per hour, or the higher your sweat rate.

So why is this so bad? When you lose sodium, your blood plasma becomes less concentrated—more watery, so to speak—than the cells in your tissues, so water moves out of your bloodstream and into your cells to even things out. Your cells swell, and the swelling of the cells around your brain causes the symptoms of hyponatremia. In addition to mental confusion and loss of awareness, you may experience headache, nausea, muscle cramps, and swelling in your fingers and toes.

What to Do

You are not likely to come across a little old man with a jar of salt during your next race, so if you do feel yourself bonking, get to the nearest water station and down a few cups of a sports beverage until you feel better. If that doesn't do the trick, search out some salty foods, like pretzels, peanuts, or, my favorite, Goldfish crackers! If there happens to be some pickle juice, go for it! Pickles and their juice are a terrific source of sodium.

Prevention

The key here is to know yourself (this not only works for sodium but also for life). In terms of sodium, everyone has a different sweat rate. It's almost counterintuitive—the fitter you are, the more you sweat. This is because your body is like a fine-tuned car, the sweat evaporating off your skin cooling the body much like a radiator cools a car. The other key point: Everyone sweats different amounts of salt (sodium). This tends to be a fixed variable; some people are "salty sweaters" and some aren't. If you look like a human deer lick, with white powder caked on your skin after a run, you are a salty sweater!

Putting this all together: If it's a hot and humid day, and if you are in good shape, and if you are a salty sweater, you will need to preload plenty of sodium with salty foods before a long workout or race. My key—be prepared! Bring pretzels on your run, buy some sodium tablets at your local running store, and make sure you hit the sports drink regularly instead of water to keep your sodium levels high.

If you start getting muscle cramps, if your stomach is upset, or if you are getting dizzy, it's probably low sodium. Hit the salt! Make sure you deal with it early since hyponatremia that isn't recognized just gets more and more serious. I have included it here as a minor malady since most cases just result in cramps, but low sodium can sometimes be fatal. Pay attention, please.

BRUISES

One of the potential hazards of trail running, a bruise usually looks uglier than it feels. With a little TLC, it will disappear fast.

What to Do

1. Apply ice for 15 minutes a day several times during the first 2 days.
2. Gently rub vitamin K cream or arnica gel (both available at your local pharmacy) into the bruised area for a few days following your mishap to speed healing.
3. To help move blood out of the bruised area, apply heat and elevate your injury above your heart.

Prevention

If you bruise easily, you may be vitamin C deficient. Vitamin C helps to build protective collagen around the blood vessels in your skin. Eat more citrus fruits, melons, berries, bell peppers, tomatoes, and leafy green vegetables.

BUNIONS

I'm going to dispel the myth about bunions once and for all. This protuberance at the base of your big toe is *not* caused by shoes that squeeze your forefeet, as most people believe. You can thank your mom or dad, or both: Genetics determines whether or not you will develop bunions. An inherited poor foot structure is the underlying cause of this progressive condition, which starts out with your big toe leaning in toward your second toe, throwing the joint at the base of your toe outward. Loose joints and tendons in your foot and the shape of your metatarsal bones all contribute to instability in the joint and allow your toe to become misaligned.

Now, here's where your footwear comes into play. Picture a high-heeled pump with a narrow, pointed toe—stilettos, sexy for sure, until you take them off. The shape of the shoe combined with the pressure of your body weight falling farther forward on your foot when you wear pumps pushes that big toe inward and puts a lot of pressure on the outward-leaning bones at the joint. Over time, that irritated joint becomes deformed, and you've got one painful bony bump at the base of your toe.

Bunions are 10 times more common in women because of fashionable shoe choices (which today have reached an all-time high in both style and potential for causing orthopedic damage), but other factors come into play, so guys, I hope you are still reading this. Flat feet and low arches cause overpronation. Keep in mind that as you push off during running, the last part of your foot to leave the ground is your big toe. So if you have an unstable joint at the base of that toe and your foot rolls too far inward as you run, you are going to push that big toe toward the second one. Finally, whether you are a woman or a man, any shoe with a narrow toe box spells bunion trouble if your foot is prone to this deformity.

What to Do

1. Wear shoes with a wide toe box that doesn't put pressure on the bunion, or consider cutting a hole in your running shoes around the bunion to relieve pressure.

2. Covering the bunion with moleskin or a gel-filled pad (available at your local pharmacy) may also help relieve pain.

3. Use an over-the-counter orthotic to control pronation.

4. For bouts of pain, take an anti-inflammatory, such as ibuprofen or naproxen.

5. To reduce swelling, apply ice for 15 minutes several times throughout the day.

6. If your bunion causes constant discomfort, see your doctor. Surgery, called a bunionectomy, might be an option, but in general I recommend that runners stay away from surgical treatment unless they have tried absolutely everything else first. The surgery to correct a bunion deformity doesn't always work, especially in runners who want to keep running.

Prevention

Bunions will progressively get larger, so the sooner you recognize you have one, the better.

- Wear footwear that doesn't squeeze your toes or put pressure on the joint at the base of your big toe.

- If you overpronate, wear over-the-counter orthotics to correct your foot motion. I love heat-moldable inserts, and there are lots of options online.

CHAFING

This ranks up there with the most annoying of the annoying runner's maladies. Whether it's skin rubbing against skin or skin rubbing against the band of your sports bra or running shorts, that friction heats things up (think rubbing sticks together to start a fire). Your chafed skin becomes red, inflamed, and may even be rubbed raw. It will certainly *feel* like it's on fire.

What to Do

Gently clean and dry the area. If it's bleeding, use hydrogen peroxide; then apply antibiotic ointment and an adhesive bandage or sterile gauze and tape.

Prevention

- Apply a lubricant to any and all vulnerable spots. There are a variety of products, including petroleum jelly, which will reduce friction. You can find them at your local drugstore or running shop. You may need to try a few different products to find what works best for you.

- Wear clothing made from synthetic, moisture-wicking fabric that helps keep your skin dry. Choose sports bras with smooth seams.

CHAFING OF THE NIPPLES

If you have been a spectator at the finish of a marathon, you may have seen a male runner come through with two red streaks running down his singlet. You guessed it—it's blood from his nipples having been rubbed raw against his shirt. Ouch! Unfortunately, this is not an uncommon experience among male distance runners. Women who wear sports bras are generally protected from this horror.

What to Do

1. When you feel your nipples chafing against your shirt, take your shirt off if you can. If that's not an option, you can pull your shirt away from your nipples, but clearly this isn't the most efficient way to run, and if you are competing in a race, you will probably choose to endure the discomfort to the finish.

2. After the race, clean your chafed nipples with hydrogen peroxide, which will, yes, sting like crazy and might incite you to spew some not-for-print language. Next, apply some antibiotic ointment and cover your wounds with an adhesive bandage or gauze secured with tape.

Prevention

I have one word for you—protection. You can try using a waterproof adhesive bandage across each nipple, but sweat might make them come loose. I have found that some of the newer soft-fabric products work better. If you want the gold standard for those monster male nipples that are tough to protect, I recommend NipGuards. These bad boys are small, round adhesive pads that cover your nipples. You should be able to find them at your local running store. Pack a few extras in case they come off in the middle of your run or race.

CHAPPED LIPS

Running in desertlike air makes a desert of your lips. Dry summer days, winter winds, and arid climates (think Arizona) suck the moisture right out of you, leaving the thin skin of your lips dry and cracked. And no one will want to kiss those babies.

What to Do

1. In the middle of a run, when you feel your lips getting dry, rub your finger along the side of your nose; you will pick up some of your skin's natural oil. Rub that into your lips.

2. At home, apply petroleum jelly, a terrific moisturizer, or your favorite lip balm.

Prevention

- Protect your lips from the elements by applying lip balm before you head outside. I like those with natural ingredients like olive oil, shea butter, almond oil, and beeswax.

- Drink plenty of fluids daily. A well-hydrated body means well-hydrated lips.

- Nutritional deficiencies can leave lips vulnerable. Make sure you are getting enough iron and B vitamins—most abundant in and absorbable from meat. A lack of unsaturated fatty acids in skin tissue may also lead to chapped lips. Eat more fatty fish, like salmon, rich in omega-3s, or consider popping a supplement daily.

COMMON HEAD COLD

I love to run. I run every day, and there is almost nothing that stops me, including a head cold. If you feel like hitting the road, go for it. But remember my rule: If you have symptoms below the neck or a fever over 100°F—stay home.

What to Do

1. Use a nasal rinse or neti pot to clear your nasal passages.

2. Drink plenty of fluids to loosen congestion.

3. Don't skimp on sleep; it's essential to keeping your immune system strong.

4. If you have a sore throat, gargling with warm salt water (¼ to ½ teaspoon dissolved in 8 ounces of water) can ease the discomfort.

5. Try vitamin C to reduce your cold symptoms. It won't cure your cold, but it might help you feel a little better.

6. Sucking on zinc lozenges may shorten the length of your cold, but if you are also taking vitamin C, take the supplements at least an hour apart since they bind together, which makes them less effective. Also, cap your zinc intake at 40 milligrams a day; more can cause nausea, dizziness, or vomiting.

Prevention

Regular running powers up your immunity. There is plenty of data showing that runners have fewer illnesses than sedentary people, so keep doing what you do, and follow this commonsense advice.

- Stay committed to your healthy lifestyle. A nutritious diet, enough sleep, and good hydration all support a healthy immune system.

- Wash your hands regularly during peak cold and flu season. And keep your hands away from your face; germs can hop into your eyes, nose, or mouth, where it's warm and moist and they can have a crazy-good time.

DEHYDRATION

Let's hope you never get dehydrated, because you drink plenty of water every day. But perhaps you have been super busy and barely stopped to take a sip of anything, or maybe you are taking a medication that has a diuretic effect, meaning it causes you to urinate frequently. You can lose a lot of water over a long run or marathon, especially when it's hot and you are sweating buckets— and if the well isn't full, it will go dry.

As I described earlier, the fitter you are, the more you sweat. When you are super fit, your body's sweat response is fine-tuned. Sweating is your body's cooling system: As sweat evaporates, your body cools down, and the more you sweat, the cooler you will be (even though you won't look cool). A problem arises, however, during a hot and humid day—you keep sweating and sweating, but since the air is humid, sweat doesn't evaporate well, and your body temperature keeps rising. The combination of heat and humidity together is called the heat index. When it's high, you are particularly prone to overheating.

Signs that you are dehydrated include thirst, dry mouth, infrequent urination and dark urine when you do go, headache, and muscle cramps. Severe dehydration can make you dizzy and light-headed, cause rapid breathing and a rapid heartbeat, and even lead to unconsciousness.

What to Do

Drink water or an electrolyte beverage immediately. If you are severely dehydrated—if you feel light-headed or have a rapid heartbeat—have someone take you to the ER; you may need to have fluids administered intravenously. If things get really rough, call 911.

Prevention

You know what I am going to say here: Drink plenty of water every day. My rule is this: When your urine is

pale yellow—I'm talking almost clear—you are getting enough fluids.

- During a half or full marathon or a longer race, take fluids at the water stops, especially when it's hot.

- If you can plan your long training runs so they will take you past public places, like parks, that have water fountains, that's great. Otherwise consider purchasing a hydration belt system or backpack so you can carry water or a sports beverage with you.

- During periods with a high heat index, prevention means more frequent fluid breaks, more electrolytes in the form of sports drinks or electrolyte tabs, and, most of all, better awareness about dehydration. I always tell my patients that it's much easier to prevent dehydration from happening during a race than to play catch-up when fluids get low and you are moving and sweating.

STEP INTO MY OFFICE

Blipp this page to view a video about dealing with various ailments that can and often do arise on race day.

DIARRHEA: RUNNER'S TROTS

Let's be honest—many of you have had to poop when you are running. Does it happen sometimes? All the time? Let's talk about it so we can hopefully put it behind us.

What you eat and when you eat come into play, but no one really knows what causes diarrhea during running. One theory is that as your

blood is diverted from your digestive tract to your working muscles, your body stops absorbing nutrients from food still in your intestines and at the same time isn't reabsorbing the water in your colon. Diarrhea by definition is the speedy passage of undigested food through your intestines before your body has reabsorbed water. When you feel the urge, you know what to do—head for the nearest restroom, portable toilet, or tall bush.

Prevention

For some, a case of runner's trots is a one-time experience, maybe the morning after a dinner of bean burritos and margaritas; you can clearly ID cause and effect. For others, diarrhea may frequently ruin long runs and marathons and the reason isn't so obvious. Experimentation is key to finding a solution.

- Keep a food journal and look for a pattern between what you have eaten and the effect on your digestive tract. High-fiber foods—such as beans, fruits, veggies, and whole grains—move more quickly through your intestines. Sugar alcohols found in sugar-free gum and candies and lactose—the sugar in milk—can cause diarrhea. Try limiting a few or all of these foods a day or two before a long run and see what happens.

- Experiment with the timing of meals and snacks. Plan for at least 2 to 3 hours between a meal and a run.

- Go ahead and have a prerace snack before your marathon, but, again, experiment with different foods, energy bars, or gels in training first. Don't try anything new on race day.

- Dehydration can cause diarrhea, so down plenty of water and sports drinks but avoid caffeinated beverages, which have a diuretic effect and stimulate bowel movements in some people.

- If you have an important event coming up and you are really concerned, you can take an antidiarrheal, such as Imodium, but try it out in training first. Also, these drugs are an occasional fix, not a long-term solution. Don't take them regularly.

- If you feel you have tried everything and you still can't rein in runner's trots, see your doctor to rule out an underlying problem.

FOOT ODOR

Here's a fun fact to throw out to your friends at your next party: Your feet and hands have a higher concentration of sweat glands than any other part of your body—about 3,000 per square inch of skin, which for the average foot comes to 250,000 sweat glands in total. (Okay, maybe you only want to share that at a runners' gathering.) So you can imagine that trapped inside socks and shoes, mile after mile, those glands release a lot of sweat. All that moisture mixes with the bacteria on your skin. It's a foot-odor cocktail that after 10, 12, 20 miles or more can get pretty potent.

What to Do

Soak your feet in either a black tea or vinegar solution for 30 minutes a day for a week, advises the American Academy of Podiatric Practice Management. This will kill the bacteria and shrink the pores on your feet. To make the black tea solution, steep two bags of tea in a pint of just-boiled water; then add 2 quarts of cool water. For the vinegar solution, combine 1 quart of vinegar with 2 quarts of cool water.

Prevention

- Always wear socks with your shoes.
- Wash your feet every day and dry them thoroughly.
- Dust your feet and the inside of your shoes with a nonmedicated foot powder.
- Have two pairs of running shoes of the same make and model so that you can alternate between pairs, allowing them to dry out completely before your next run.

HEAT EXHAUSTION

Heat illness is a spectrum of problems, from the benign and self-limited heat cramps all the way to the sometimes-fatal heat stroke.

Let's start this discussion with the term *heat index*, which is a measure of what the temperature feels like when humidity and air temperature are combined. The higher the heat index, the hotter you feel, the bigger the strain on your body's cooling system, and the greater your risk of heat illness. You can significantly lower your risk of

heat illness with the following three strategies.

1. Acclimatization—gradually adapting to running in hot and humid conditions
2. Good hydration
3. Recognizing the early stages of heat illness so you can head off its progression

Now let's take a look at the stages of heat illness.

MILD HEAT INJURY

At this early stage, you will experience cramps in your stomach or in your muscles that fire as you lose fluid and salt.

What to Do

1. Stop running.
2. Stretch your muscles to relieve the cramps.
3. Drink cool water or a sports beverage that is low in sugar.

181

MODERATE HEAT INJURY (AKA HEAT SYNCOPE)

This is when loss of fluid and salt leave you feeling weak, tired, and dizzy. You may even feel faint.

What to Do

1. Stop running and seek out a cool, shady area.

2. Drink cool water or a sports beverage that is low in sugar.

3. Place a cool, wet towel or cloth around your neck to help you feel better.

HEAT EXHAUSTION

Now things really start heating up (pun intended). You have been sweating buckets, but now perspiration is starting to decrease as your skin and body temperature rise. Symptoms include thirst, extreme fatigue or weakness, muscle cramps, dizziness, confusion, headache, nausea, vomiting, and pale, clammy skin.

What to Do

1. Stop running and seek out a cool, shady area.

2. Ask for assistance from another runner or race personnel.

3. Drink cool water or a sports beverage that is low in sugar.

4. Apply cool, wet towels or cloths to your body.

HEAT STROKE

At this point, your body temperature is probably over 103°F. Your skin is hot and red and could be moist or dry. You may experience nausea, vomiting, confusion, or dizziness. Unconsciousness is possible.

What to Do

1. This is a medical emergency. Call 911.

2. Get immediate help and get to a cool, shady place.

3. Do *not* drink fluids.

4. Place cool, wet cloths over your skin.

Prevention

- I have three words for you: hydrate, hydrate, hydrate. You know you are drinking enough fluids when your urine is very pale.

- Give yourself time to adjust to heat and humidity. When spring turns to summer or you head to Florida for the winter, cut back on mileage and intensity and build back up gradually over a period of 7 to 10 days.

- Run during the coolest times of day and wear light clothing.

- When it is really hot and humid, check the heat index and adjust your running accordingly. Don't go too far or too fast when the index is high, and consider taking your run to a treadmill in an air-conditioned gym.

- Know the signs of heat illness, and if you run or race under hellish conditions, listen to your body. Stay aware, and if you notice even mild symptoms, call it a day so that you have many more days ahead of you to run. My take-home points for exercising in the heat: be safe, be mindful, and be smart. Heat illness is 100 percent preventable if you take care to recognize the symptoms early and head them off at the pass.

INGROWN TOENAILS

Here's justification for getting regular pedicures—ingrown toenails. You don't want them. If you trim your nails incorrectly, they can grow into the skin of your toes, and it's painful. The area turns red and tender. And running with an ingrown toenail? As with any other foot pain, it's no fun.

What to Do

1. Use an over-the-counter product to soften the skin and nail. Choose one like Dr. Scholl's Ingrown Toenail Pain Reliever or Outgro Pain Relieving Liquid, which contain an anti-inflammatory ingredient to help ease the discomfort. Apply according to the package directions.

2. Soak your foot in warm salt water (use 1 teaspoon of salt for every pint of water) for 5 to 10 minutes three to four times a day. Dry your foot, and then take a thin piece of sterile cotton or waxed dental floss, apply some antiseptic, and insert it between your ingrown nail and the skin. This will help the nail grow past the sore skin. Change the cotton or floss daily.

3. Wear sandals or shoes with a roomy toe box to keep pressure off your toe.

4. If your toe swells and becomes redder and more painful or if you see a discharge, your toe may be infected. See your doctor, who will treat the

infection and then may recommend partial removal of the nail.

Prevention

- Cut your nails straight across, not in a curve, and don't cut them too short.

- Wear shoes that give your toes the space they need. Shoes that are too tight in the forefoot can also cause ingrown toenails. Make sure there is a thumb's width of space between the end of your longest toe and the top of your running shoe.

MUSCLE CRAMPS

You are running along and suddenly you experience a sharp gripping in your muscle that feels like it's never going to let go. It can be painful enough to pull you over to the side of the road. Your quadriceps are the usual victim of muscle cramps, but calves are not immune.

A nutritional deficiency, dehydration, lack of sodium, and muscle

DODGING LYME DISEASE

You're achy, tired, and feverish. You feel like you've got the flu, but it's spring. Cold and flu season has passed. What's going on?

You may have Lyme disease, a bacterial infection whose early symptoms resemble those of the flu. Make an appointment with your doctor if you think you have Lyme, because the sooner you treat it, the more effective the antibiotics will be in clearing it up completely. Lyme disease is transferred to humans by deer ticks in their nymphal stage—when they are young and tiny—making them difficult to see. The first symptom is a red rash that looks like a blotch or a bull's-eye (a red spot surrounded by clear skin and then a ring of red), and it is quickly followed by fever, chills, achy joints, and fatigue. If you experience these flulike symptoms, check for a rash, but even if you don't find one, see your doc, especially if you have been running on trails, in the woods, or through high grass or live in the Northeast or Upper Midwest and it is any season but winter. If a blood test comes back positive for Lyme, your doctor will prescribe antibiotics.

How to dodge it: When you are headed for a trail run, dress for defense and wear socks that come up above your ankles. Don't head off-trail into the woods or brush, where you are more likely to meet up with deer ticks. As soon as you get home, peel off your clothes and check them for ticks, and then search your body, keeping in mind that deer tick nymphs are tiny—the size of a pinhead. Ticks seek out cozy hiding spots, so be sure to check behind your knees, in your groin area, and around your neck.

If you do find a tick, use a pair of fine-pointed tweezers, grasp the little bugger as close to your skin as possible, and pull firmly and directly outward. Place the tick in some rubbing alcohol to kill it. Clean the bite with an antiseptic, such as hydrogen peroxide; then watch the area for any signs of rash or other symptoms, which can appear anywhere from 3 to 30 days after a bite.

fatigue all can cause a muscle to become a little "edgy." The muscle anticipates a contraction and then simply contracts on its own. Cramps occur most often at the end of a race, when your muscles are fatigued and depleted of water or key nutrients.

What to Do

1. Slowly stretch the contracted muscle. Go gently and gradually. When one muscle cramps, another may follow. When you stretch your quad, for example, you simultaneously shorten your hamstring. To prevent a reciprocal cramp, be careful not to contract your hamstring; focus on keeping your whole leg relaxed.

2. Drink lots of fluids.

3. Rarely do cramps require a doctor's attention, but if you get them chronically despite your best efforts to prevent them, make an appointment with a physician, who will work with you to determine whether the cause is nutritional or functional and will prescribe a plan to help you find relief.

Prevention

- Strengthen your muscles to help prevent fatigue at the end of a race. Do the IronStrength workout once or twice a week (see Chapter 12 and watch the videos), and if you are still prone to quad cramps, add in some squats and lunges.

- Use your foam roller regularly. Lack of flexibility also makes you prone to cramping.

- Stay well hydrated. You will know you are if your urine is pale.

- Eat a well-balanced diet to make sure you get all the nutrients you need, and in hot, humid weather, salt up your diet the day before a long race or run; add a little salt to your spaghetti, or have some pretzels. And drink electrolyte beverages on the run to replace sodium lost in sweating.

STEP INTO MY OFFICE

Blipp this page to view a video about prevention and treatment of cramps.

NAUSEA AND VOMITING

Here's another unsightly finish-line image to rank up there with bloody T-shirts from chafing: A runner goes all out in a 5-K, pushing it to the limit, squeezing out every ounce of effort to beat a competitor or break a PR; steps across the finish line; and vomits on the side of the road.

Nausea and vomiting can also happen at the starting line when race-day jitters jostle the contents of your tummy.

PRERACE

When you are nervous or anxious about competition, adrenaline rises, which is a good thing because it powers your performance. But rising adrenaline causes blood to be redirected away from your digestive system to your muscles as they get ready to work. Consequently, your gastrointestinal tract can't function as it normally does and stops moving food from your stomach into your intestines. If your prerace jitters have also created tension in your abdominal muscles, the pressure just might push the contents of your belly up and out.

Prevention

- Two days before your race, switch to a low-fiber, low-fat diet. Cut back on fruit and high-fiber cereals; no bran muffins. Choose foods that are easily digested—pastas, white rice, bagels, bananas. And don't eat anything for at least 2 to 3 hours before your race. If you do need to eat a snack—before a marathon, for example—grab something light and quickly digested (see Chapter 15 for more tips about prerace fueling). Please test prerun eating in training; don't try anything new on race day. I'm a huge fan of applesauce race morning. It goes down easy, rarely comes back up, and tastes great.

- Sip a sports drink or take an energy gel 30 to 45 minutes before the gun goes off. This will regulate your blood sugar at the start of the event.

- Don't let anxiety get the best of you. Establish a prerace routine that can focus your mind on preparing to run your best, including a warmup; channel that anxiety into positive actions for success (see Chapter 14 to learn how to master your mind-set for peak performances).

MIDRACE

During exercise, your body's priority is to direct blood to working muscles that are in need of oxygen and glucose for energy production. So with less blood flowing to your gastrointestinal tract, the flow of food slows down. Whatever is still in your stomach, instead of moving down into the small intestine, might come up.

Prevention

- Experiment with what and when you eat as described above to find what your digestive system can tolerate during racing.

- Try not to take an anti-inflammatory before your race; they have been linked to vomiting during endurance events.

- If you eat sports nutrition bars or gels before or during a race, follow up with water, not an electrolyte beverage, which will deliver another shot of sugar. Too much sugar in your belly can make you queasy.

POSTRACE

Vomiting after a race—particularly after a hard, fast effort for which you busted your gut in a sprint to the finish—may be the result of the sudden, rapid drop in physical exertion. Though the rest of your body has stopped moving, your stomach may still be contracting.

Prevention

Though you may not want to move another step after your fastest 5-K, try to jog or at least walk slowly to gradually bring all your body's systems down together.

SIDE STITCHES

I have never met a runner who hasn't experienced side stitches, though I would say it's most common among new runners. You will feel this cat-and-mouse pain in your side; it comes on while you're running and may force you to stop. When you do stop, the pain goes away, only to return once you start up again.

Side stitches usually signal a diaphragm spasm. Your diaphragm is the muscle that separates the lung and chest cavity from the abdominal cavity. When your diaphragm contracts, it moves downward, opening up the chest cavity, which allows the lungs to expand and bring in air. As your diaphragm relaxes, air is pushed out of your lungs. When you are running, your diaphragm is working hard, and if you don't have enough core strength to support your working diaphragm, it will get angry and go into spasm. This is why stitches are more common in beginning runners who have not yet built up running-specific strength.

What to Do

1. Try to relieve the side stitch while running. Raise your arm on the side that hurts, and place your hand on the back of your head. This stretches your obliques (muscles on the sides of your chest). Hold this position for 30 to 60 seconds. Repeat if the pain doesn't stop or if the stitch returns.

2. If that strategy fails, try this: Stop running and stretch the muscles in your side by bending to the opposite side of the stitch.

3. If side stitches are chronic and nothing you do provides relief, see a sports doctor. The pain may indicate a lung-related issue, such as exercise-induced bronchospasm (aka exercise-induced asthma) or an anatomical abnormality with your lungs. With either diagnosis, your doctor will prescribe an inhaler.

SUNBURN

I have spoken to several groups of runners over the years, and I can usually pick out the ones who have been doing this for a long time because they look a little weather-beaten. Listen, it's not that I care about a few wrinkles; I care about your health. Dermatologists I have spoken with tell me that the number of cases of sun-related cancers they have treated has grown tremendously in the past several years. If you are fair-skinned and have light-colored hair and blue or green eyes, you burn more easily than most, and with every deep and painful sunburn you get, you increase your risk of developing skin cancer. According to the Skin Cancer Foundation, if you have had five or more sunburns in your lifetime, your risk for melanoma—the deadliest of skin cancers—doubles. So I will tell you about how to manage a wicked sunburn, but more importantly, let's then talk about how you're *not* going to get burned.

Prevention

Since the most common cause of side stitches is muscular, do the Iron-Strength workout once or twice a week (see Chapter 12 and watch the videos) and get in some extra core-strengthening exercises, such as planks and crunches, throughout the week.

What to Do

1. Take a cool bath to soothe your skin or soak some washcloths in cold water and lay them over the burn. You will feel the washcloth get warm after several minutes. Replace it with a fresh, cold cloth.

2. Take an anti-inflammatory, such as ibuprofen or naproxen, to help ease the pain.

3. Apply moisturizer, aloe vera gel, or hydrocortisone cream. Do not use petroleum jelly or other oil-based products, which can clog your pores and prevent heat and sweat from escaping. Also, do not use benzocaine or other "-caine" products; they may irritate the skin or cause an allergic reaction.

4. If blisters form, don't break them; simply cover them with a dry bandage.

5. Drink plenty of water to rehydrate.

CANINE ENCOUNTERS

When you come home after a long day to your pup bounding toward you—tail wagging, tongue lolling—it's a happy sight. When a strange dog comes at you on your run, that's a scary one. Most dogs would rather chase a groundhog than a human, but then you run by and trigger the canine prey instinct, and before you know it, Cujo is nipping at your heels.

If a dog you don't know starts running toward you, walk. If he comes right up to you, stand still, sideways to the dog, and stay as calm as you can. Watch out of the corner of your eye, but don't look the dog in the eye, which he will take as a sign of aggression. In most cases, the dog will lose interest and walk away.

Still standing there? Invoke the mojo of Cesar Milan: Use your biggest, deepest, most authoritative "I am the boss here" voice and tell the dog to "Go!" If the dog believes you are the one with the power, he will leave.

But let's face it—none of us is Cesar Milan. So if your big stance doesn't send the dog on his way and he starts growling and baring his teeth, you need to switch to protection mode. Give the dog something to bite other than your arm if you can—a sweatshirt, hat, anything. It might distract the dog enough that you can retreat to a safe place. Otherwise, cross your arms over your chest and make fists with your hands, using them to protect your neck. Yell for help. If you are bitten, resist the urge to pull away because the dog's teeth will make trenches in your flesh.

If you have been bitten: Wash the wound with soap and water as soon as you can. For a scrape, apply an antibacterial ointment, such as bacitracin. Clean the wound once a day, and if you see redness, swelling, and drainage, you probably have an infection and need to get it treated by a physician.

If the dog punctured your skin, try to find out if he is up to date on rabies shots and then head to your doc or the ER, depending on the severity of the bite. You may need a tetanus shot or a series of injections to prevent rabies.

Finally, report the incident to your local police. Rabies or not, a dog that bites you might bite others. Your local authorities will keep track of the number of incidents and take further action if needed.

Prevention

- Thoroughly slather a waterproof broad-spectrum (protects against UVA and UVB rays) sunblock with a minimum SPF of 30 over every exposed inch of skin. Use a shot-glass-size dollop of cream (2 tablespoons, or 1 ounce) 20 minutes before you head outside. If you are using a spray, apply enough to create an even sheen over your skin. Most docs have found that creams are more effective than sprays, so that is what I recommend you use.

- Sunscreen should be reapplied every 2 hours, and more often if you are sweating profusely. If you plan to be out for a few hours, place some in a small plastic bag and carry it in your shorts pocket. The sunscreens containing zinc (read the back of the bottle) tend to work best, so try those first.

- Wear a hat to prevent your scalp

from getting burned, and consider sun-protective clothing.

- Wear sports sunglasses to protect the skin around your eyes.

- The sun is strongest between 10 a.m. and 4 p.m., so try to plan your runs for early morning or early evening.

URINARY INCONTINENCE

The uncontrollable leakage of urine during running is the bane of many female runners, particularly those who run during pregnancy, when the growing uterus puts pressure on the bladder. Then there's childbirth, which can weaken or damage the muscles and nerves needed for bladder control. Stress incontinence occurs when a physical action—such as coughing, sneezing, or exercise—increases the pressure within the abdomen and your weakened muscles can't hold the urine back.

Prevention

- Avoid drinking caffeinated beverages, which increase urine production.

- Until you have regained full bladder control after childbirth, wear a light absorbent pad.

- Strengthen the muscles of your pelvic floor by doing Kegel exercises. Squeeze the muscles you would use to stop urine flow. The challenge with Kegels is knowing whether you are using the right muscles. If there's a pulling-up feeling when you squeeze, you are using the right ones. Also, you should not be using the muscles in your abdomen, butt, or thighs. When you first start doing Kegels, lie down so that you don't have to work against gravity. Squeeze for a count of three, and then relax to a count of three. Work up to 3 sets of 10 repetitions daily. It may take 3 to 6 weeks to see improvement, so hang in there.

- If after 6 weeks there is still no improvement, see your doctor. He may recommend a pessary, which is a stiff ring that you insert into the vagina, where it puts pressure on the vaginal walls and the nearby urethra to prevent leakage. Your doctor may also discuss injections of bulking agents, such as collagen, into the tissues around the urethra and the neck of the bladder to reduce the bladder opening and prevent incontinence. And finally, surgery may be recommended to reposition your bladder.

YEAST INFECTION

Three out of four women will have at least one vaginal yeast infection at some point in their lifetimes. A yeast infection is an irritation of the vagina and vulva. Yeast is a fungus that is always present in the vagina, but when it grows to excess, it causes an infection. You will suffer, and I mean suffer, extreme itchiness in and around the vagina and may also have to endure one or more of the following symptoms: burning; swelling; redness; a thick, white discharge that looks like cottage cheese; and possibly pain during urination and sex. Several factors increase your risk for a yeast infection, including stress, lack of sleep, pregnancy, and eating way too many sugary foods. Runners are vulnerable because of all the heat and sweat generated during a run that is then trapped inside their shorts.

What to Do

See your doctor to confirm a diagnosis. She may recommend an over-the-counter antifungal cream or ointment or prescribe a dose of oral fluconazole. Be sure to let your doctor know if you are pregnant since that will determine the best and safest course of treatment.

Prevention

- Don't use douches.
- Wash with water and a perfume-free, pH-balanced soap, like Dove.
- Change out of running shorts as soon as you can.
- Wear cotton underwear during the day and no panties at night to allow good airflow, which helps moisture evaporate.
- Limit your time in hot tubs.
- Eat yogurt that contains *Lactobacillus acidophilus* regularly, daily even. It helps maintain healthy levels of bacteria and fungi in your vagina.
- Take antibiotics only when necessary; they kill off the good bacteria with the bad.

PART III

Getting the Most from Your Machine

How do you build and maintain a great body that stays healthy and injury-free and runs really well? This is what I call getting the most from your machine. It makes a huge difference for every runner reading this book, beginner to elite.

CHAPTER 12
BODY WORK

Running does a great job of developing certain muscles—your calves, hamstrings, and quads, for example. But others—including your glutes, hips, and core—don't see a lot of action yet are super important to stability. Then there's your upper body, which is mostly just along for the ride, but your arm swing balances your leg swing and your upper-back and shoulder muscles help out with stability. So you might have five-star quads, three-star glutes, and one-star shoulders.

Our modern sit-on-your-butt lifestyle makes muscle imbalances even worse. Maybe you run an hour a day every day, but that still leaves a lot of hours to sit: during your commute, in front of the computer at the office, around the dinner table, in front of your favorite TV show. Your hamstrings and quads aren't crazy about this because while you're sitting, your hams are flexed and your quads are stretched, and over time your hamstrings become tighter and your quads weaker.

Muscular imbalance is one of the big reasons runners get injured, but it is easily corrected. The solution is two-fold.

- Build your whole body with strength training.
- Use a foam roller every day over your whole body to loosen up tight spots and keep all your muscles supple.

This is probably the stuff you're not doing, but it's going to do amazing things for your body.

The IronStrength Workout for Runners

If you are like most of the runners I meet in my office, you are probably not strength training. Seriously—I will see someone for a hip problem and suspect they're not doing any strength training, and when I ask, the answer is almost always no. Strength training is one of the most important things you can do to build a healthy kinetic chain and prevent injury. I recommend at least one and preferably two dedicated strength sessions per week.

I began developing my IronStrength workout after wandering into a functional strength-training class run by my good friend Dejuana Richardson at Asphalt Green, a fitness center in New York City, 6 years ago. I was looking for something to help me manage the arthritis that started burning in my knee 15 years after I tore my ACL playing soccer. I found it in functional strength training—working your muscles using real-world movements. For my IronStrength workout for runners, I took that real-world concept further with exercises that mimic running movements. Since running is a one-leg-at-a-time activity, you will see lots of single-leg exercises in this workout. I also love plyometrics, which rapidly elongate and contract muscles, similar to what you do when you run. And of course, since your goal is balanced strength up and down your kinetic chain, IronStrength is a total-body workout: It hits your lower, middle, and upper body. Plus, while each exercise targets certain muscles, your whole body gets involved, just like it does when you run.

IronStrength isn't easy. I don't mess around. I want you to work hard, and I set the bar high for each exercise. But I also want you to approach it from your own level of fitness. If you can do every move at the goal right out of the gate, great. If you need to do fewer reps, fine. If you want to make it harder, shorten the rest between sets. Adjust the workout to your level of fitness, and build as you get stronger.

The IronStrength workout for runners is total-body, real-world training that works your muscles with running-specific movements. Commit to it twice a week, and I promise you will be really happy you did. Let's get started.

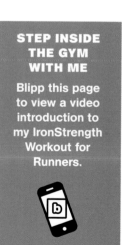

STEP INSIDE THE GYM WITH ME

Blipp this page to view a video introduction to my IronStrength Workout for Runners.

THE DYNAMIC WARMUP

Going into a strength workout cold is not a good idea. It puts a lot of force on a body that is not prepared for the physical demands of the workout. You need to get your muscles, joints, and bones moving; your blood flowing; and your brain ready for action. A lot of people like to stretch before a workout, but here's what static stretching does—lengthens muscle and tendon, and that's about it. It doesn't increase bloodflow, and it doesn't wake up the neuromuscular pathways that you will be firing once you start using your muscles.

A better way to go is a dynamic warmup that gets everything moving, including your heart. A dynamic warmup says to your brain, "Hey, muscles have been flexed, joints are rolling, blood's delivering food and oxygen, we're ready to rock and roll." Another big benefit to a dynamic warmup is that it gets your muscles working both concentrically and eccentrically. With concentric contractions, your muscles shorten as they contract. For example, your quads contract and shorten to extend your knee and lower leg as you prepare to land during running. With eccentric contractions, your muscles lengthen as they contract. That seems like a contradiction, right? So let's look at an example. One of your hamstrings' jobs during running is to control your leg during landing. As your leg straightens out before footstrike, your hamstrings are stretched as they contract to prevent too much forward motion.

A dynamic warmup moves muscles in all ways—lengthening, contracting, and doing both at the same time.

So for this warmup, I would like you to do 30 seconds of jumping jacks, 30 seconds of squats, and 30 seconds of lunges to get your body ready for the "heavy lifting."

WAIT! WHAT ABOUT STRETCHING?

Stand at the starting line of any race and you will see runners staggered-stance to stretch their calves, bent over a straight leg to loosen hamstrings, or pulling a leg back to lengthen their quads. Prerun stretching is a running ritual that began and continues with the belief that it will prevent injury. Research, however, hasn't really supported that belief. In fact, one study found a *higher* incidence of injury when runners stretched before a workout.

That same study noted a lower rate of injury among runners who stretched *after* their run. Stretching definitely relaxes muscles after a hard effort, so save it until you have crossed the finish line of your race or workout. There is an increasing amount of information that foam-rolling might be even more effective than stretching, so some runners are only rolling these days. My take is that both are helpful, but if you're going to do only one, I'd prefer you roll.

JUMPING JACKS

Stand with your feet together and your hands at your sides. Simultaneously raise your arms above your head as you jump your legs wide out to the side. Immediately reverse the movement and repeat.

Why you do them: Jumping jacks get your whole body moving, but they especially wake up your calves, hip abductors and adductors, shoulders, and core. And they rev up your cardiovascular system.

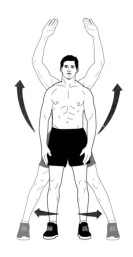

SQUATS

Stand with your feet about hip-width apart. With your arms straight out in front of you, slowly lower down as if you are going to sit; push your butt back and engage your core to keep your upper body upright. Lower until your leg forms a 90-degree angle, and then push back up. Repeat.

Why you do them: Squats target your quadriceps, hamstrings, glutes, and core.

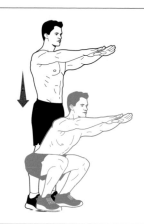

REVERSE LUNGES WITH A TWIST

Stand tall with your arms at your sides. Lunge back with your left leg until your forward (right) leg is bent about 90 degrees. As you lunge back, raise your left arm and twist your body and arm to the right (the side of the forward leg). Push back to standing, and then lunge back with the opposite leg. Repeat, alternating legs. Keep your upper body upright, and don't let your forward knee move beyond your toes.

Why you do them: Lunges get your quads, hips, and glutes moving, and the twist brings your obliques into the action. You will also use your core muscles for stability and balance.

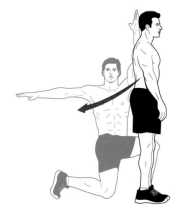

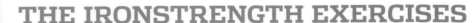

THE IRONSTRENGTH EXERCISES

Once you have completed the dynamic warmup, you can dive into the following exercises. You should feel warm all over, maybe a little sweaty. I recommend listening to great music for the upcoming strength work. It really helps! Do the exercises in the order presented here; I alternate lower body, upper body, lower body, upper body. And please watch the videos. Seeing these moves performed properly will help you follow in good form and get the most out of each exercise.

STEP INSIDE THE GYM WITH ME

Blipp this page to view a video demonstration of a proper plyometric jump squat.

① PLYOMETRIC JUMP SQUATS

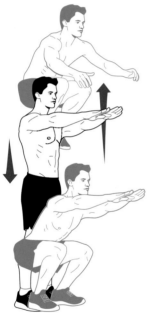

I always say the key to a happy running life is a strong butt. When you have a strong butt, your hips are happier and your knees are happier. Squats are a great way to strengthen your butt. I like to start with these because they are really hard and they work your muscles and your cardiovascular system.

Stand with your feet spread a little wider than shoulder-width and turned out just a little bit. This helps you get low. Put your arms straight out in front of you. Now lower down until your butt is just below your knees. As you lower, push your butt back, as if you are going to sit down in a chair, and keep your torso upright. Explode up off the floor, and then come right back down into the squat. Repeat.

Points for good form: Use controlled motion, landing softly each time, and push off from your heels as you come up.

Reps: Do 6 sets of 15, with 20 seconds of rest in between. You can build up to 8 sets.

Modification: If you can do plyometric jump squats but you can't do 6 sets of them, that's okay. Do what you can and build up to 6. If plyometric squats are too hard, do isometric squats. It's the same exercise, just don't come up off the floor.

THE RIGHT WEIGHT

You will need weights for a few of the IronStrength moves. I suggest beginning with hexagonal dumbbells, which have flat sides on each end for better balance. As you become more adept with these exercises, you can switch to rounded dumbbells, which are more difficult. For women, I recommend 6- to 8-pound weights; for men, 10 to 15 pounds.

SUPERSET: ROWS FROM PLANK, PUSHUPS, SITUPS

A superset is a combination of exercises, and in this case, I have combined three moves for your core and upper body.

STEP INSIDE THE GYM WITH ME

Blipp this page to view a video demonstration of a proper superset of these exercises.

ROWS FROM PLANK

Planks are great for strengthening your core, and rows rotate your core and upper body simultaneously.

Get into a plank position with your hands resting on dumbbells. Your spine should be straight, shoulders over your hands, feet hip-width apart, and core engaged. Pull the left dumbbell up next to your chest, and then lower it down. Repeat with the right arm. You don't want to turn your whole body; you should still be basically facing the floor. Do 15 (left and right equals 1), and then move on to pushups.

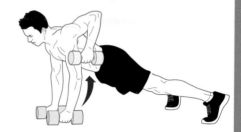

PUSHUPS

Pushups have been around forever, right? And for good reason: They're simple and they strengthen your core and upper body.

Get into a plank position (spine straight and core engaged), lower your body almost all the way to the floor, pause, and push up. If your hips start to droop, switch to a modified version. Do 15, and then flip onto your back for situps.

Modification: I would like you to do as many traditional pushups as you can. When you feel your butt start to sag, though, drop to your knees but keep your spine straight and your core engaged as you lower your upper body and push back up.

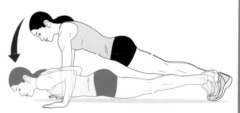

SITUPS

Situps are another old-school exercise that is good for the core—your abs specifically.

Lie down on your back with your knees bent, feet flat on the floor, and hands behind your head.

Come off the floor, sit straight up, and lower back down.

Do 15 reps; then begin the superset again with rows from plank.

Duration of the superset: I would like you to spend 5 minutes on this superset, 6 minutes if you're advanced.

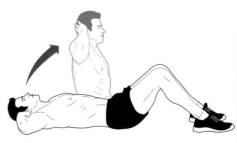

③ SUPERSET: PLYOMETRIC LUNGES AND SINGLE-LEG TOE TOUCHES

Back to the lower body now, with two exercises that are great for your lower legs and your glutes and work your body in ways that specifically relate to running.

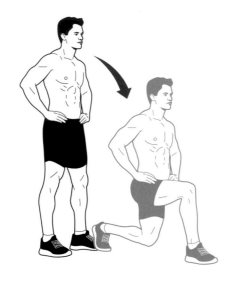

PLYOMETRIC LUNGES

These are really hard, but what I love about them is that they mimic running motion. When you run, you shift your weight from one leg to the other, and that's what you are going to do here.

Start with a simple isometric lunge:

From a standing position, lunge forward with your right leg and left arm, lowering your body until your back knee nearly touches the floor. Engage your core muscles to keep your torso upright and stable. Push back up and repeat with your other leg.

Build in plyometrics:

Perform the lunge as described above, but as you come up, really push off the floor so you can switch legs in mid-air. Then immediately come back down into the lunge and explode up again.

Points for good form: Accentuate the leg movement; your legs should be farther apart than they would be if you were running. Engage your core; you want very controlled motion and a stable pelvis—no flailing around. Come on, you know you're having fun now! Right?

Reps: Do 10; then move on to the plyometric single-leg squats.

Modification: Your goal should be to do plyometric lunges for the entire set. If you can do that on day one of this workout—terrific. If you can't, stick with isometric lunges and gradually work in the more advanced plyometric version as you are able.

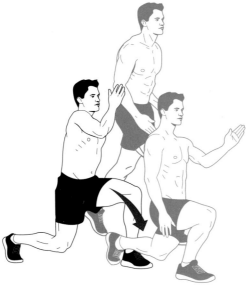

SINGLE-LEG TOE TOUCHES

These work your glutes, the top of your hamstrings, and your core, and they improve balance and stability.

Start with an isometric single-leg toe touch:

Stand on your right leg with your left leg out in front of you and raised off the floor. Place your arms straight out to the side at shoulder height. Bend your right leg at the knee and squat down to touch your left hand to the toe of your right foot; then come back up.

Build in plyometrics:

Perform the exercise as described above, adding in a hop as you come back up.

Points for good form: Engage your core to keep your torso upright and control your movement as you lower your body.

Reps: Do 10 on your right leg; then go back to the lunges. For your second superset, do 10 on your left leg.

Modification: The goal is to do plyometric single-leg toe touches throughout the entire set, but these are really challenging. Please don't get discouraged. Perform the isometric toe touch as best you can, and if you can't touch your toe, that's okay; just reach down as far as you can comfortably while maintaining good form.

Duration of the superset: Alternate between the lunges and toe touches for a total of 5 minutes, 6 minutes if you are advanced.

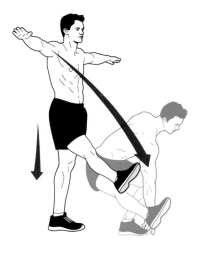

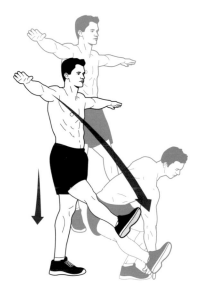

STEP INSIDE THE GYM WITH ME

Blipp this page to view a video demonstration of proper plyometric lunges and single-leg toe touches.

STEP INSIDE THE GYM WITH ME

Blipp this page to view a video demonstration of a proper mountain climber and legs down.

④ SUPERSET: MOUNTAIN CLIMBERS AND LEGS DOWN

This terrific superset really works your core and your cardiovascular system. You will feel like you climbed a mountain after you've done this set.

MOUNTAIN CLIMBERS

Your abs and glutes get a great workout when you do mountain climbers, and your heart rate will climb high too.

Get into a modified straight-arm plank position with your butt a little higher than if you were doing planks. Bring your right leg forward as far as you can—your knee will come close to your arm—and then immediately extend it straight back and bring your left leg forward. Switch back and forth quickly from leg to leg.

Points for good form: Maintain the modified plank position throughout; don't let your butt sag or poke upward. Your upper body should be stable; all the movement happens from the hips down.

Reps: Right and left counts as 1; do 15, and then flip on your back for legs down.

Modification: You can make these easier by supporting your upper body on a bench or exercise step.

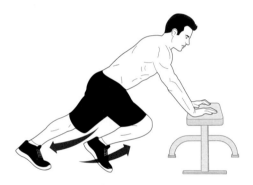

LEGS DOWN

This exercise is harder than it looks. It builds a ton of core strength as your muscles work against gravity.

Lie down on your back, legs straight and together. Keeping your legs straight, bring them all the way up and reach for the ceiling until your butt comes off the floor. Slowly lower your legs back down almost to the floor, and then raise them back up again.

Points for good form: Use controlled motion throughout the exercise, raising and lowering your legs slowly.

Reps: Do 15; then return to mountain climbers.

Duration of the superset: Repeat for a total of 5 minutes, 6 if you are advanced.

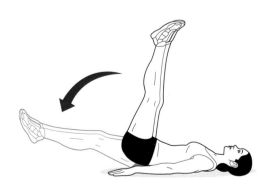

⑤ SUPERSET: DEADLIFT HIGH PULLS, OVERHEAD PUSH PRESSES, BICEPS CURLS

Here we are going to focus on your upper body, which is important to runners for stability and balance.

DEADLIFT HIGH PULLS

These will strengthen your glutes, the top of your hamstrings, and your lower back.

Holding a dumbbell in each hand, stand with your feet shoulder-width apart. Squat down about 30 degrees, sticking your butt out and keeping your back straight. Hold the dumbbells straight down by your knees with your palms facing back. Stand up and pull the dumbbells up next to your ears in a nice fluid motion, and then lower back into the squat position and repeat.

Points for good form: Maintain fluid motion as you squat down and pull up.

Reps: Do 15; then get ready for the overhead push press.

OVERHEAD PUSH PRESSES

I like to have you stand on one leg while you do this move and the bicep curls (up next) so you make your core work to keep you balanced while you exercise your arms.

Standing on one leg, hold a dumbbell in each hand right above your shoulders with your palms facing in toward your ears. Push the dumbbells straight up and come right back down, using your core to keep your balance.

Reps: Do 15; up next—bicep curls.

Modification: If you have trouble balancing on one leg, try just touching your toe to the floor for a little stability.

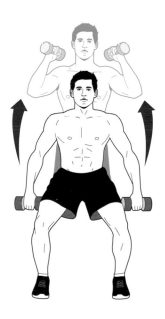

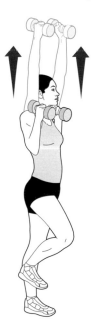

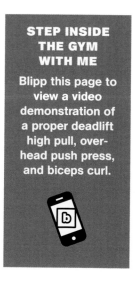

STEP INSIDE THE GYM WITH ME

Blipp this page to view a video demonstration of a proper deadlift high pull, overhead push press, and biceps curl.

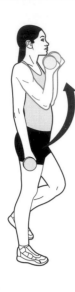

BICEPS CURLS

Again, balancing on one leg while you do these works your core while you build your biceps.

If you stood on your right leg for the overhead push press, I want you to now balance on your left. Hold a dumbbell in each hand straight down by your legs, palms facing forward. Curl both dumbbells up toward your shoulders, and then release them back down. Repeat using a nice fluid motion.

Reps: Do 15; then start from the top of the superset again with deadlift high pulls.

Modification: If you have trouble balancing on one leg, touch the toe of your raised leg to the floor for some stability.

Duration of the superset: Continue to rotate through the three exercises for 5 minutes, 6 minutes if you're advanced.

---

⑥ BURPEES

Also known as squat thrusts and the jail-cell exercise, burpees have been evaluated as the most difficult exercise you can do. They use just about every muscle in your body and require strength, power, and endurance—of muscle and mind. You are going to hate these, but as you get better, you will learn to like them, I promise. If you don't hate me when you're doing your burpees, you aren't working hard enough.

Stand with your feet shoulder-width apart. Squat all the way down, placing your hands on the floor. Supporting your weight on your hands, kick back into a plank position. Do a pushup. Pull your legs back into a squat, and then jump straight up in the air.

Points for good form: Be sure to hold your torso upright and push your butt back as you lower down into a squat. And kick into proper plank position, straight body from heel to head; don't let your hips drop or stick up.

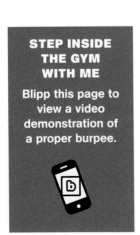

STEP INSIDE THE GYM WITH ME

Blipp this page to view a video demonstration of a proper burpee.

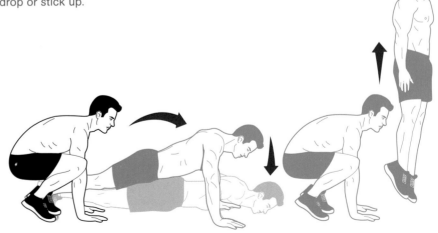

Reps: Do 4 or 5 sets of 10 (yes, that's 40 to 50 burpees in total), with 20 seconds of rest between sets. Once you get really good at these, I want you to do a burpee pyramid, descending from 10 sets of 10 to 9 sets of 10, then 8, 7, 6, all the way down to 1 (no kidding).

Modification: I really want you to conquer this exercise, and I know you can do it. But if you need to start out with a modified version, that's fine; there are a few different ways to change it up and make it easier. If you can't do a traditional pushup, do the pushup on your knees. If the squat-and-thrust portion is giving you trouble, use an exercise bench or step and instead of going all the way to the floor, support your body with your arms on the bench as you kick back and then do the pushup. Do what you can and build on it, and when you can finally do full-out proper burpees, send me a tweet!

THE FINALE: PLANKS AND STRETCHING

We're going to finish up with some planks and some static stretches for your whole body. Though I don't like stretching before a workout when you are cold, now that you're warm, stretching is a good way to relax muscles and prevent them from tightening up after an intense workout.

PLANKS

These are terrific core builders, and you can do them every single day.

Start with a right forearm plank: Lie on your right side and support your body on your forearm, elbow directly under your shoulder. With your left arm pointed straight up to the ceiling, raise your hips until your body is in a straight line from your shoulders to your ankles. Hold this position for 1 minute. Turn facedown to do a center plank; support your body on both forearms, elbows directly under your shoulders, and engage your core muscles to hold your body in a firm line from head to heel. Hold steady for 1 minute. Turn to your left to finish with a left forearm plank, holding this final position for 1 minute.

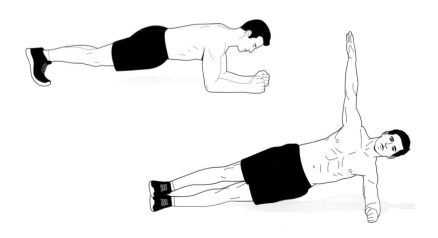

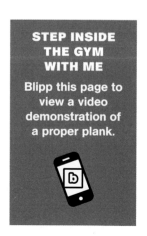

STEP INSIDE THE GYM WITH ME

Blipp this page to view a video demonstration of a proper plank.

Now let's stretch all those muscles that you have worked so hard today.

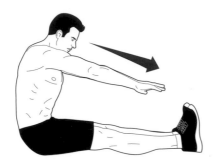

SEATED HAMSTRING STRETCHES

Sit down on the floor with your legs together and straight out in front of you. Lean forward toward your feet, stretching out your lower back and hamstrings. Don't worry about trying to touch your toes; go as far as you can comfortably and hold for 15 to 20 seconds. Next, spread your legs apart a little and bend toward your right foot; hold for 10 to 15 seconds. Then bend toward the left for 10 to 15 seconds.

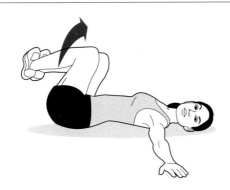

BACK STRETCHES

Lie on your back with your legs together and bent. Keeping your shoulders on the floor, move both legs together over to your right as far as you can go without lifting your shoulders off the floor. Hold for 15 to 20 seconds; then twist and take your legs over to your left side, again as far as you can go without lifting your shoulders, and hold for 15 to 20 seconds. This stretches the erector spinae muscles located along your spine.

MODIFIED PIGEON POSES

Face the floor, fold one leg underneath your upper body, and stretch the other leg straight behind you. Lean forward as far as you can comfortably and hold for 15 to 20 seconds. This stretch really opens up your glute muscles. Switch legs and stretch the other side for 15 to 20 seconds. As you become more flexible, you will be able to bend farther forward.

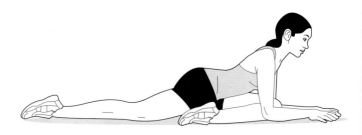

HIP FLEXOR STRETCHES

Your hip flexors are a group of muscles in the front of your hip that flex your hip and bring your thigh up toward your chest. You worked them hard during lunges, mountain climbers, and burpees. To stretch them, get down on the floor, bring your right leg forward a little bit in front of your knee, and extend your left leg behind you, knee resting on the floor a little bit behind your butt. Stretching your arms up over your head, arch your back as you lean into your forward knee. Hold for 15 to 20 seconds, and then switch legs.

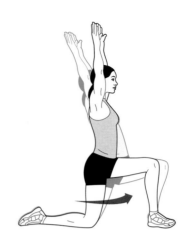

ACTIVE OBLIQUE STRETCHES (AKA I'M A LITTLE TEAPOT)

Stand tall with your feet shoulder-width apart. Take your right arm and stretch it all the way up as high as you can toward the ceiling. This stretches the obliques and all the muscles along the side of your rib cage. Hold for 15 to 20 seconds, and then stretch the other side.

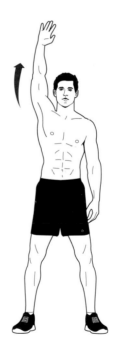

Congratulations, you have completed the IronStrength workout for runners. It will take about 50 minutes. Schedule it twice a week—at least once. I promise you will be just as thrilled with the results as runner Dail St. Claire is. (You can read her story on page 216.)

THE FULL-BODY FOAM ROLLER ROUTINE

A healthy kinetic chain also needs balanced flexibility throughout—full range of motion from heel to head so one tight muscle isn't pulling everything out of whack. Let's say you have tight hamstrings. Your hammys attach to the top of your pelvic bone, so when they are tight, they pull down your pelvis, which makes your lower back flatten out and inhibits those muscles from contributing to stability. So the psoas muscles kick in, but they're not stability specialists, and they tire quickly and get strained.

How do you balance flexibility? For years runners and other athletes have used stretching to keep muscles loose and free of injury, and there is a time and a place for stretching. But when it comes to day-to-day flexibility conditioning, nothing beats the good old foam roller.

You probably know about the foam roller if you don't already have one. It's a cylinder about 6 inches in diameter made of dense foam. You can get one in a sporting goods store or online, and you will find lots of options. Which is best? Choose the one that feels right for you and that you will use every day. They generally range in size from about 12 to 36 inches. If you think you will be rolling both legs at the same time, choose the longer roller. I like the hollow ones with a softer outside. If you can, test out the rollers at your gym or ask your friends if you can try theirs.

Now, if you don't have one, stop reading this book, try a couple versions, and buy or order one. Then I want you to make a commitment to use it every day. This simple piece of equipment is going to become your body's best friend. Let's look at what the foam roller can do for you and how to use it to care for every major muscle group in your body. Your body will thank you.

I mentioned earlier in the book how important regular massage is for healthy muscle tissue. Well, the foam roller is like a massage—one that you give yourself. By rolling your hamstrings, quads, and glutes back and forth over this hard foam cylinder, you loosen muscle and fascia—the thin layer of connective tissue that wraps around and in between muscle and bone and other tissues. Foam-rolling can release an adhesion—a spot where muscle and fascia are stuck together. It promotes bloodflow and relaxes muscle and fascia to allow the range of motion you need to prevent injury and run your best.

I have to warn you that it's going to be uncomfortable at first, and if you have a particularly tight muscle or an adhesion, rolling that spot is going to hurt. But that pain is your muscle crying out for help, letting you know it's too tight and needs some relief. Plus, the payback is that postworkout muscle soreness will be diminished. As you regularly roll your muscles and unwind those tight spots, foam-rolling will become less painful. Eventually, you will enjoy it, and you definitely won't miss the trouble that a tight calf or hamstring causes you.

Here are three guidelines before we get started.

- Roll slowly back and forth for about 30 seconds.

- Don't roll bony areas, such as the side of your knee or the side of your hip; stop just above or below these spots.

- If you hit a tender spot, stay on it for 30 to 90 seconds, despite the fact that you will be grimacing in pain. Trust me, it's good for you.

Now, let's roll!

HAMSTRING ROLLS

Position the foam roller under your right hamstring just above your knee, and cross your left leg over the right at your ankle. Place your hands flat on the floor for support. Now roll your body forward until the foam roller reaches your butt. Then roll back until the roller reaches your knee. Continue to roll back and forth; then repeat on your left side.

Note: Crossing one leg over the other puts more weight on the hamstrings as you roll them and may cause too much pain. In that case, simply uncross your legs and roll both at the same time.

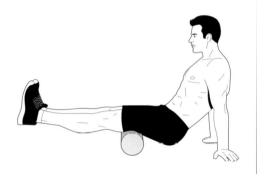

GLUTE ROLLS

Sit with the foam roller positioned at the top of your right hamstrings, just below your glutes. Your knees should be bent and your feet flat on the floor. Now cross your right ankle over the top of your left thigh, and place your hands flat on the floor behind you for support. Roll forward on your glutes until the roller reaches your lower back; then roll back and forth. Switch sides to roll your left glute.

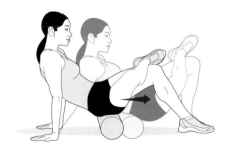

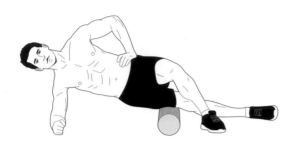

ILIOTIBIAL BAND ROLLS

I am going to be honest with you, a lot of runners find this exercise pretty uncomfortable. The iliotibial band (IT band) is a fibrous band of tissue that runs along the outside of your thigh from your hip to just below your knee. In runners in particular, it can get kind of tight, especially in those who overpronate or have weak hip muscles. A tight IT band can cause trouble for your knee or hip, so you definitely want to roll it regularly. If it's tight, it's going to hurt, but as you continue to roll it, the discomfort will slowly disappear.

Lie on your right side with your right hip on the roller. Lean on your right forearm for support. Cross your left leg over your right and place your left foot flat on the floor. Roll your body forward until the roller reaches your knee; then roll back and forth. Repeat on your left IT band.

CALF ROLLS

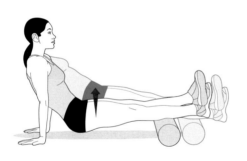

Position the foam roller under your right ankle, and with your legs straight, cross your left ankle over your right. Place your hands flat on the floor beside you and support your upper body on your arms as you roll your body forward until the roller reaches the back of you knee; then roll back and forth. Repeat with your left calf.

Note: Crossing one leg over the other puts more weight on your calf as you roll it and may cause too much discomfort. In that case, simply uncross your legs and roll both at the same time.

QUAD ROLLS

This move will also create flexibility in your hip flexors.

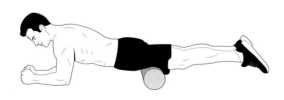

Lie facedown on the floor with the foam roller positioned above your right knee, supporting your upper body on your forearms. Cross your left leg over your right at the ankle. Roll your body backward until the roller reaches the top of your right thigh; then roll back and forth. Repeat with your left leg.

Note: As mentioned with previous foam roller exercises, if it hurts too much to roll one leg at a time, roll both legs at the same time.

GROIN ROLLS

Lie facedown on the floor with your foam roller placed parallel to your body on the right side. Support your upper body on your forearms. Bend your right leg to the side and rest the area of your inner thigh near your knee on the foam roller. Now roll your body to the right until the roller reaches your pelvis. Roll back and forth, and then repeat on your left side.

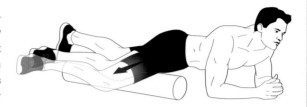

UPPER-BACK ROLLS

Lie faceup with your foam roller under your upper back at the tops of your shoulder blades. Cross your arms over your chest, bend your knees, and place your feet flat on the floor. Raise your hips and roll up until the roller reaches your mid-back. Roll back and forth over your upper back.

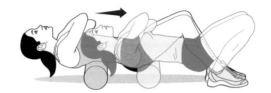

LOWER-BACK ROLLS

Lie faceup with your foam roller under your mid-back, knees bent and feet flat on the floor. Place your hands on the floor for support. Raise your hips off the floor slightly and roll up until the roller reaches the top of your glutes. Roll back and forth over your lower back.

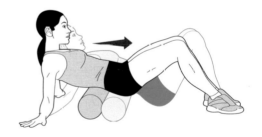

I would love for you to foam-roll your muscles before and after you run, and your muscles would love that too. But I get it that your schedule just might not allow it. (You really should get back to your desk and do some work after your lunchtime run.) The good news is you will get all the great benefits of foam-rolling any time you do it—even while you're watching tonight's episode of *The Late Show*. No excuses.

Rashid Naseem: One with the Universe

Running, for me, is a prayer, a meditation.

I don't compete. I run because of the way I feel when I run. My thinking mind shuts down and my body takes over, moving in sync, creating the act of running. And I am totally aligned with my surroundings. My feet can feel the paint on the road in Central Park, my body can sense approaching cyclists on the bike path, my ears can pick up the different languages in Time Square. I'm not running but flowing. I'm one with the universe.

Five years ago, I couldn't run at all. I even developed trouble walking because of acute pain in my right foot. The first doctor I consulted suggested that I might have a hairline fracture that couldn't be picked up in an x-ray. So I went to see Dr. Metzl, and he diagnosed a pinched nerve—Morton's neuroma. He gave me a cortisone shot in my foot, and I was fine the next day.

Then there were my knees. I always had pain in my knees when I ran. I went to a running store, where they watched me run on a treadmill and told me that I overpronate. They recommended a stability shoe and then I started running, increasing my mileage little by little.

Three years later I ran the New York City Half-Marathon, and then I signed up for the New York City Marathon lottery and was selected. Unfortunately, Hurricane Sandy cancelled the race. The following year after a visit to Istanbul, I decided to enter the Istanbul Marathon, which crosses the Bosphorus Bridge, connecting Europe and Asia.

As the universe would have it, the announcement came for the New York City Marathon and the date was only 2 weeks before Istanbul. Dr. Metzl advised me not to do both, but how could I not run the New York City Marathon? It was in my hometown.

Every day for 2 weeks prior to New York, I used the foam roller, following Dr. Metzl's program in *The Athlete's Book of Home Remedies*, and I had very little pain or stiffness after the marathon. I continued to use the foam roller every day prior to the Istanbul Marathon. I carried it (and my Pilates mat) to Istanbul and religiously used it. People looked at me rather quizzically. But I ran another successful marathon—the foam roller saved me.

I had finished New York in 4 hours and 30 minutes and then Istanbul in 4 hours and 45 minutes. I was supremely proud of myself for running 52.4 miles in just over 9 hours in two countries across three continents in 2 weeks. And I was fine afterward. In fact, I walked 4 miles to get back to my hotel after the Istanbul Marathon and spent the next day strolling along the Bosphorus.

Today I run as much as I can, and I usually do at least one long run each week. Running gives me a lot of stamina. It brings balance to my life, both physically and emotionally. I can't imagine my life without it.

MASSAGE: PUTTING YOUR MUSCLES IN THE HANDS OF A MASTER

If you foam-roll every day, why would you ever need another massage? Great question. Rolling and massage both apply pressure to loosen tight muscles, undo adhesions (spots where muscle and fascia stick together), and speed recovery. The difference is that you and your foam roller don't have nearly the expertise or the touch of a massage therapist. Don't get me wrong, I love foam-rolling and do it every day— but it's kind of like the difference between giving your partner a back rub with your bare hands and using boxing gloves.

When a massage therapist kneads your muscles, he *feels* what's going on—the tight tissue, the malleable muscle—and can determine how far to push and when to lighten up. A therapist can go in on the exact spot of those adhesions and really unstick them, and though this hurts like hell, it opens up those muscles to a full range of motion. Then there are the areas of your body where muscles aren't tight or stuck together, where massage just feels pretty darn won-

derful. Despite the moments that make you want to leap off the table, when all is done and you slowly slip off and into your shoes, you will feel soothed.

Runners, coaches, and massage therapists have been proponents of regular massage for years. Now scientists are excited to discover that massage produces some really amazing results. They were not too surprised to confirm that it restores flexibility and unties knots, but they were wide-eyed over these findings.

Massage stimulates increased production of mitochondria in muscle cells. Mitochondria are the engines of your cells, taking nutrients and oxygen and producing the energy your cells need to work and to make repairs. Researchers believe this bump in mitochondria is at least in part responsible for speeding recovery after a long or intense workout, which in turn lessens the intensity and duration of delayed onset muscle soreness and lets you get back to hard training sooner.

THE MYTH OF MASSAGE THERAPY

For decades, athletes, coaches, and therapists have believed that massage pushes toxins and lactic acid out of your muscle, hence the healing effect—an interesting idea, but scientifically untrue.

It improves immune function. Emory University researchers measured higher numbers of several types of lymphocytes—white blood cells that fight infection—in muscle after just one massage.

It reduces inflammation. The Emory study also found that massage decreased levels of cortisol in the blood. Cortisol is a hormone that rises during stress and has been linked to chronic inflammation throughout the body. Unlike acute inflammation, which very noticeably causes pain and swelling, the chronic systemic version lays low. You likely won't even know it's there, and yet it can be deadly, contributing to the development of serious ailments, including cardiovascular disease and cancer.

Bottom line: Massage improves your health as a runner and a human being. The bonus: It can help you achieve better running performance. I give it two thumbs up and recommend you try to get in two massages each month in addition to daily foam-rolling.

Dail St. Claire: Iron Woman

My friends call me Forrest Gump.

At the age of 50, I walked/ran my first half-marathon, and I haven't stopped running since.

I saw Dr. Metzl a few months after the half, not for a running injury but because I had sustained whiplash from a car accident. After treating my whiplash, Dr. Metzl asked if I wanted to join in his Iron-Strength workouts. He said to think of it like fortifying the framework of a building—I would be strengthening the infrastructure of my body. So I joined.

I couldn't do most of it when I started, but I went at my own pace, and eventually I saw a change in my body. I was stronger. The day I could do pistol squats without falling over is a day I will never forget.

Every year I run two marathons, and I have even qualified for Boston. I have learned that with all the miles, you have to build strength. It makes you a better runner. I do IronStrength at least once a week and twice a week when I'm training for a marathon—with 18-week marathon training periods a year, that is 36 weeks of training and 64 IronStrengths during those periods. And guess what? I am running injury-free.

I have embarked on this adventure called running, and I want stay on it for the rest of my life. So I think I will stick with those IronStrength workouts too.

SLEEP: THE NEGLECTED SUPERHERO

We have been talking about what you can do to build a strong, flexible, healthy body that resists injury and performs at its best. Well, here is the easiest and one of the most effective things you can do—sleep. Sleep builds strength, and the hardest effort you will have to put forth is the commitment to making time for it.

When you are awake, your body is busy supporting everything you do, from eating a club sandwich to working at your computer to reading a book, going for a walk, doing the dishes, digesting your club sandwich— you get the point. When you're asleep and not doing any of that stuff, your body can shift its attention and energy to the internal tasks of cleanup, repair, and rebuilding. Truth is, scientists haven't been able to uncover exactly what's happening in your body during the night shift, but they do know it's busy in there. Neurotoxins are neutralized. Growth hormones are released. Cells divide. And your body builds new bone, muscle, tendon, and other tissue where it's needed. Learning that occurred during the day gets locked into your brain and unnecessary info is swept away. A lot happens in the night to help you feel refreshed and ready for a new day when you wake up in the morning.

A good night's sleep is restorative. Sleep deprivation can be deadly. Studies show that those who sleep fewer than 6 hours a night have a higher risk for obesity, heart disease, diabetes, and poor brain function. And sleep on this: Researchers at the University of Surrey in England took blood samples from 26 people who slept for 10 hours a night for a week; then they asked those same 26 to cut their sleep to fewer than 6 hours a night for a week. Again, blood samples were taken, and the researchers discovered that the drop in sleep had altered more than 700 genes. So, what does all that mean? The specifics are still being explored, but it's not pretty. Sleep deprivation impairs your immune system and weakens your body's ability to bounce back from stress and damage.

Kind of makes you want to hit the

SLEEPLESS BEFORE RACE DAY?

Don't worry about it. Studies show that one sleepless night does not ruin running performance.

Declines don't begin to show up until after two nights of tossing and turning.

sack right now, doesn't it? Well, if it's 10 p.m. and you have to get up at 6 a.m., you might want to do just that. Seriously, lock in 7 to 8 hours a night. Here are some tips for how to get the sleep you need.

- Go to bed and wake up at the same time every night and day, even on the weekends.

- Skip the nightcap. Alcohol might make you feel sleepy, but it will disrupt your sleep throughout the night.

- Choose decaf if you like a cup of coffee after dinner.

- Exercise helps you fall asleep and improves sleep quality, but don't work out within 3 hours of your bedtime.

- Ban TVs, tablets, laptops—anything with a screen—from the bedroom. A busy mind and the blue light emitted from these devices make it harder to fall asleep. Use your bedroom for sleep and sex only.

- Keep your room dark, quiet, and a comfortable temperature.

- A regular nighttime ritual signals your brain that it's time to shut down and catch some shut-eye.

Life is crazy-busy. I get that. But putting in the sleep hours you need at night pays you back in awesome performance during the day—at work, at home, and on the road, running. Sweet dreams.

CHAPTER 13

REV IT UP: Mastering the Science of Running Physiology

I've given you my Rx for building a strong, healthy body:

IronStrength once or twice a week
+ Foam-rolling daily
+ Massage once or twice a month
+ Sleep 7 to 8 hours every night

The next piece in your injury-prevention plan is to *use your body right*. Train smart. Build a schedule that follows the rules of healthy running, because when you break the rules, you break down. And when you break down, you can't train. And when you can't train, you won't improve as a runner, whether your goal is a fun 5 miles of running every other day or to race your fastest 5-K ever.

USE IT RIGHT

A quick review: The main causes of overuse injury are muscular imbalance, mechanical stress, and training errors. Strength training and flexibility work take care of muscular imbalance and help you manage mechanical stress, but the real solution to preventing stress and overuse injuries is smart training.

Rule No. 1: Don't Do Too Much Too Fast

It's the old (really—it's been around for decades) 10 percent rule, which goes like this: Increase your mileage no more than 10 percent each week.

When you ask your body to do something it's not prepared for—either your body hasn't yet learned the job or the workload is way too heavy—*stress injuries* occur. Muscle tears, strains, and stress fractures are typical stress injuries. Let's say you are a marathoner and someone challenges you to a 60-meter sprint. Your muscles aren't trained to produce explosive movement. Sprinting shocks the system with a sudden and heavy load, and the probability for failure and injury are high. Same goes for the sprinter who hasn't done any long-distance running and enters a marathon. It's a different kind of load—a load of miles on muscles and bones that aren't ready for it, and the consequences can be disastrous. These are extreme examples, for sure, but you get the point: Asking too much of a body that's not prepared for the job is asking for injury.

Preparation isn't defined by only your level of strength and fitness. You need *specific* fitness. The marathoner in the above example may be strong and cardiovascularly fit, but not for sprinting. You need to prepare specifically for the kind of running you want to do, whether that's shorter and faster or longer and slower. And as with anything you do, there is a learning curve. Running—any movement—is neuromuscular; your muscles respond to complex nerve impulses sent by your brain down neural pathways. These impulses travel faster than you or I ever could. Still, you need to teach your brain to find the best pathways, and you want to reinforce those pathways by using them again and again in training.

Rule No. 2: Build Rest into Your Training

Follow hard days (long miles, speed-work, hill repeats) with easy days. When I say use those neural pathways again and again, don't go crazy because then you might succumb to an *overuse injury*. The phrase defines the malady. Running is by definition repetitive motion: You hit the ground over and over again in the same way mile after mile. But if you don't take a break to recover from the action, *you* will break. Most running injuries are over-use injuries—Achilles tendonitis, stress fractures, knee injuries, iliotibial band syndrome. These don't happen suddenly like a muscle tear or a sprained ankle; they happen over time through repeated stress to the bone or muscle. And though correcting muscle imbalance helps tremendously in preventing these types of injuries, you also need to follow a training plan that allows you to rest and rebuild. No matter how fit you are, physical activity causes trauma to muscle and bone—and that's a good thing; it's part of the strength-building process. But you only get stronger when you allow your body to regroup and recoup, repair damage, and rebuild stronger. It's why sleep is so important. But you also need to build rest into your training. Here's what happens when you don't.

Let's say you feel great—strong, rested, no aches and pains; I'll give you a body score of 10 out of 10. You go for a fast-paced 10-miler and pound that score down from a 10 to a 4. You get a good night's sleep. Your body does some repair work, and you're back up to an 8 in the morning. Then you go for another 10-miler, this time over crazy big hills, and you knock your score down from an 8 to a 2. Sleep gets you back up to a 6 by the morning. The next day you have scheduled an interval workout—you can see where this is going. By building rest days into your training, which might be a day off from running or a slow 5-miler, depending on your goals, you allow your body to fully recover, making you much less vulnerable to injury. You will also enjoy training a whole lot more.

Rule No. 3: Listen to Your Body

Training plans are built around how many miles you should run each week and what pace you should average on your long runs, how many intervals to do and how long and how fast. Please, don't make running a numbers game. Numerical guidelines are just that—guidelines. Even the 10 percent rule is a

REFRESHER COURSE

The three main causes of running injury are:
- Muscular imbalance (strength and/or flexibility)
- Mechanical stress
- Training error

guideline, not a commandment set in stone. Some runners may increase their mileage by 10 percent and get hurt; others may be able to handle a bigger increase. Training is individual. How will you know what's right for you? Listen to your body. Pay attention to pain. If you have just bumped up your mileage and your knees hurt when you run, back off until you can run comfortably again and then slowly increase. Always remember, if you have pain during running that changes your form or the way you run, stop, walk home, and then pick up this book.

When it's hot and humid, you feel sluggish, or your usual easy 5-mile run isn't easy, slow down or cut your run short. You don't gain anything in fitness—and certainly not in fun—by pushing yourself on those days when the environment or your physiology is telling you to chill.

As you increase your training, stay alert to overtraining. This is when you have simply been going too hard day after day, week after week—too much mileage, too many hills, too much speedwork, or all of the above. You might not experience any pain, so you just might overlook this one. Here are the signs: declines in the quality of your workouts, fatigue, muscle soreness, loss of motivation, moodiness, irritability. If this is you, cut back on your training before you become injured. Consider taking a week off from running and doing some relaxed

MAX OUT YOUR MAX VO_2

What the heck is max VO_2? It is simply the maximum amount (volume) of oxygen your muscles can use when you are running as fast as possible. It is measured in milliliters of oxygen per kilogram of body weight per minute. An adult who doesn't exercise at all may have a max VO_2 of 35, and an elite marathoner may have a max VO_2 somewhere between 70 and 80. How can you learn yours? You would have to go to a physiology lab, where you would run on a treadmill while being hooked up to equipment that measures your oxygen intake as you run faster and faster until the point where you would fall off the back of the treadmill. The volume of oxygen you use at that point is your max VO_2.

For years this has been considered the gold standard for predicting running performance, but when you look at race times of elite athletes, you will find competitors who have similar race times at the same distance but vastly different max VO_2 levels. There are also those runners with similar max VO_2 levels but dissimilar performances. Go figure. Improving your max VO_2 will produce faster race times, but it doesn't mean you will beat a rival who has a lower max VO_2.

We do know that genetics influences your max VO_2 and how it will respond to training. We also know that a bigger max VO_2 is associated with bigger performance, but since oxygen consumption rises with exercise intensity, scientists are beginning to ask this question:

Does a high max VO_2 allow you to run fast, or does fast running produce a high max VO_2?

Stay tuned for the answer, and in the meantime, do some interval training to get your body to do a better job of moving and using oxygen.

swimming or cycling to keep yourself moving but allow your body time to heal. When you return to running, you will feel refreshed, energetic, and happy to be back. I promise.

Get to know yourself as a runner. It takes time, experience, and awareness. Pay attention to how you feel and work with it. The payoff will be years and years of running your best.

UP CLOSE: THE PHYSIOLOGY OF BECOMING A BETTER RUNNER

In Chapter 2, I talked about your running mechanics and form: how you run from the feet up and the best way to stack your kinetic chain for healthy, injury-free performance. Before we get into how to put together a healthy training plan, let's get under your skin and check out what's happening physiologically to get the fuel you need to your muscles so they can move.

Training is an active education not only for your muscles but also for other players in your physiology.

- Your respiratory system, where oxygen and carbon dioxide exchange takes place

- Your circulatory system—heart and blood vessels—which delivers oxygen, water, and fuel to working muscles and whisks away waste products

- Your endocrine system, pumping out hormones and enzymes that regulate delivery of glucose, uptake of glucose by your cells, fat storage, and energy production

- Your nervous system, which governs everything your body does

When these systems work together efficiently and harmoniously, you will enjoy your best running. Let's take a look at this collaborative effort.

If you are seeing me in my office in New York City and I want some more information on how I will improve your physiology, I simply refer you to my friend Polly, who runs our physiology testing center at the Hospital for Special Surgery. If you live in Anchorage, Alaska, you are probably too far to come visit us, so I will talk a little bit here about what you can do on your own.

Energy to Burn

Without energy—and I'm not talking about the "hey I'm really pumped to go for a run" kind of energy, but the kind produced along the metabolic pathways of your muscles—you aren't going to get up from reading this book, never mind hit the road. How do you create energy? First, you need fuel and oxygen—the same essential ingredients you need to make a fire.

- Your lungs draw in air.

- Your heart pumps blood to your lungs to pick up oxygen and drop off carbon dioxide (called the oxygen–carbon dioxide exchange).

- That oxygen-rich blood heads back to your heart and then is pumped to your muscles and organs.

- Circulating blood picks up glucose (fuel) and other stuff—nutrients, enzymes, hormones—and delivers all of it to your muscles and organs.

- Your muscle cells grab what they need from your blood, including the two lead stars of energy production: oxygen and glucose.

Now for the big bang.

- Glucose is broken down in a 10-step chemical process called glycolysis, and the end result is pyruvate. During this process, a little bit of ATP (adenosine triphosphate), the direct energy source for your muscles, is produced. Oxygen is usually present during glycolysis but is not essential for glycolysis to take place.

- Pyruvate then enters the mitochondria of your muscle cells for the final chemical process, called the Krebs cycle, which creates the lion's share of ATP—the energy your muscles use. Oxygen is essential for the Krebs cycle to run.

Though I have laid it out simply, the process is complex. All along the way, a bunch of different molecules, enzymes, and hormones are busy breaking down carbohydrates into simple glucose, helping to move materials in and out of your cells, escorting pyruvate into the Krebs cycle, signaling chemical reactions to keep going or to stop. Electrons get passed around, molecules are put together and taken apart—it's pretty awesome stuff.

WHAT'S BURNING? CARBS OR FAT?

You are always burning carbs, fat, and protein, day and night, whether you're running, sleeping, or posting Instagrams. But the mix changes. Fat burning is slow. First, enzymes convert fat to fatty acids. The fatty acids are then transported to your muscles and taken up by your muscle cells, and finally they enter the chemical process that produces energy.

When you're watching TV and not using much energy, you burn more fat because you're not going anywhere, so you can wait around for it. When you're running and running really fast, your muscles need energy now, and glucose is in hot demand.

You become more efficient at glucose metabolism by training at high intensities, and you become a better fat burner by running long, slow distance. Through endurance training, your body learns to increase the enzymes you need to break down fat. You also build more mitochondria—the engines of energy production. And as you improve, running becomes less stressful overall: Lower stress equals lower energy consumption, so you don't need to rely as heavily on glucose for fuel.

And the mastermind behind the scenes is your brain, quietly directing the entire production: the beating of your heart, the actions of blood vessels to move blood along, the inhalation and exhalation of your lungs, the release of hormones, the contraction of muscles, and the rate at which it all happens. As your body continues to cycle through all these actions, energy is produced and you keep running, and running smoothly.

TAKING THE SHOW ON THE ROAD

So how do you get better at running? How do you make it more fun? How does it become seemingly effortless, whether you want to glide down the road for a few miles every other day or you want to put out your best effort and bust over the 5-K finish line in your best time ever? You have to work the system in three key ways.

1. Teach your body to use oxygen more efficiently.

2. Improve your lactate threshold.

3. Invest in your running economy.

The O₂ Factor

No oxygen, no energy, no running. Keep it flowing and energy flows to your muscles. Of course, the faster you run, the greater the energy demand, and the more oxygen you need. How do you get more?

- A bigger, stronger heart that can pump more blood to your muscles
- Stronger respiratory muscles that can move greater amounts of air in and out of your lungs and more efficiently move oxygen into your bloodstream
- Efficient extraction of oxygen from your blood by your muscle cells

And how is all that going to happen?

Training.

As you run regularly, your heart gets bigger and stronger and pushes a greater volume of blood through your circulatory system with each stroke. Your lung capacity expands, and the transfer of oxygen to your bloodstream becomes more efficient; the amount of plasma (the fluid that carries your blood cells) increases; your body produces more hemoglobin to transport more oxygen to your muscles; and a bigger network of capillaries grows in and around the muscle fibers in your hardworking legs. (Capillaries are those really, really tiny blood vessels with very thin walls that allow easy transfer of stuff in and out of your cells.) All of this helps deliver more oxygen more quickly to your energy-hungry muscles.

If you are just beginning to run, there's no special training you have to do for all these wonderful changes to take place. Just run. Your body adapts; it learns what it needs to do—structurally and physiologically—to function well at the level of running that you do. You will feel the transformation when it happens. On your first trip down the road, your heart will pound and you will take big breaths; it won't be comfortable. But after a while, as you continue to run from week to week, it gets easier, and one day you will find you're cruising along—your breathing is controlled and your heart pitter-patters as you click smoothly down the road.

Eventually you hit a fitness plateau; you have reached the top of the learning curve. If you want to get to the next level of running, you will need to make some changes to your training to challenge body and mind.

If you are a new runner or your goal is to run at a moderate pace primarily to maintain fitness, increasing mileage gradually is the best way, initially, to improve your body's ability to move and use oxygen. If you are a competi-tive runner and you love to race and chase PRs, you will need to inject some high-intensity (fast) workouts into your training.

Moving the Threshold

Think back to the metabolic pathway. As you need energy, glucose is broken down into pyruvate, which gets shuttled off to the Krebs cycle for the last phase of energy production. Sometimes there's a backup at the station and pyruvate ends up waiting for the shuttle. While it's waiting, an enzyme turns it into lactate, which can be converted back into pyruvate and transported to Krebs for energy production, or sent to the liver and stored as glycogen.

As you run faster, you recruit more muscle fibers. Your leg muscles need more energy. Glycolysis speeds up. More pyruvate is produced and converted into lactate as it waits to be shuttled to the Krebs cycle. If there is little oxygen in the cell, the Krebs cycle grinds to a halt and lactate really builds up. When there is too much lactate hanging around, some of it gets pushed into your bloodstream, where

ORGANIC CHEMISTRY 101: LACTIC ACID OR LACTATE?

These terms get thrown around interchangeably, but are they really the same? Almost. Lactic acid is formed from pyruvate, but because it is an acid and your body doesn't like too much acidity, a hydrogen ion is removed from lactic acid to make lactate, which is not acidic. Same goes for pyruvic acid and pyruvate: Pyruvic acid is the end product of glycolysis, but because of its acidity, it is quickly converted to pyruvate.

it flows along and is picked up by other muscle fibers or by your organs and used to produce energy; or it gets sent to the liver and is packed into glycogen for storage.

Two really important points to note here:

1. Lactate (aka lactic acid) is easily converted back to pyruvate, making it a source of fuel that can be used by muscles (including those in your legs) and organs all over your body to produce energy.

2. If too much lactate was left hanging out in your muscle cells, glycolysis would stop, which means that you would too. Excess lactate must leave your muscle cells for energy production to continue.

Lactate is not the demon runners and coaches have made it out to be all these years. *Lactate is your friend.* And here's an eye-popping fact to share at your next runner's party: Lactate is a quicker source of energy than glucose. Think about it: Lactate is just a step away from becoming pyruvate; glucose is 10 steps away.

Here's another cool, who-would-have-thought-it piece of physiology trivia: Some level of lactate is almost always floating around in your bloodstream and getting picked up by cells or taken in by the liver. But when you're exercising hard and producing lots of lactate and spilling a lot of it into your bloodstream, you begin to approach lactate threshold (LT), which

is defined as the point when the rate of lactate entering your blood rises significantly faster than the rate that lactate is being removed from your blood by other muscle cells, tissues, and organs. And as you run above and beyond this threshold, running becomes uncomfortable. This is probably why we have considered lactate a foe for so many years. But lactate isn't the cause of your discomfort. So what is? Scientists theorize that the heat or higher acidity that occurs during the fast chemical process of energy production causes burning and fatigue.

Now, I know what you're thinking, and this is for sure the million-dollar question: When you're running hard and need lots of energy and need it fast, why the heck is lactate going to pile up? Why isn't the Krebs cycle motoring along, churning through all that pyruvate so that it doesn't even have to turn into lactate in the first place? Or why isn't the lactate being used for energy? Here are some possible answers.

- Not enough oxygen is getting to your muscle cells to work with all the pyruvate that is being produced. And that may be because your heart isn't pumping blood fast enough or you don't have enough capillaries in your muscle tissue to deliver oxygen to those energy-hungry muscle fibers.

- You may lack enough enzymes to direct all the pyruvate you have created through the Krebs cycle.

Fun Fact

Your heart loves lactate. This nonstop, hardworking organ needs a lot of energy, and lactate is a quick source.

- Your muscle cells may not have enough mitochondria to handle a huge energy demand.

- The muscle cells and tissues throughout your body that are happy to fish lactate out of your bloodstream may not be very good at pulling it up.

If you have a high lactate threshold, it means your body is expert at all of the above and you can run at a fast pace before you reach that threshold. How do you determine your LT? You could have it measured in a physiology lab, where you run on a treadmill at increasingly faster paces to exhaustion. At intervals during your run, blood samples are taken and lactate levels measured. The point in your running pace at which lactate rises steeply is your lactate threshold.

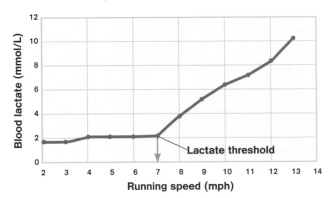

But of course, getting your LT measured in a lab costs money. A reliable way to determine your lactate threshold on your own is to run your fastest mile. Go to a track and time yourself for four laps (better yet, go with a

friend who will motivate you to run your hardest); 85 percent of your mile time is your pace at lactate threshold. The good news about your lactate threshold is that you can raise it with high-intensity training at 85 percent to 100 percent of your mile pace (more on that later).

Running Economy

We have talked about improving your body's ability to use oxygen and about raising your lactate threshold, and I hope you can see how these really are linked; we are in essence talking about your physiological chain, right? There's one more link in this chain that is perhaps the most important of all, and that is running economy.

Running economy is the amount of oxygen your body uses at a given running speed. Since oxygen and energy are directly tied, you can think of them interchangeably as I talk about running economy. For some runners, an 8-minute-per-mile pace is really difficult; it requires a lot of energy, and they use a lot of oxygen as evidenced by their hard breathing. Other runners can click off 8-minute miles while expounding on the virtues of plyometric strength training to their running buddies. These efficient runners use less oxygen. You would rather be in that second group, wouldn't you? Well, your genes will have a fair amount of input on just how fast you will be able to run on a given amount of O_2, but you *can* influence these economic indicators:

- How high you push off the ground as you run (vertical oscillation)
- Arm swing
- Stride length
- Ground-contact time
- Stability
- Number of mitochondria in your muscle cells
- Strength and efficiency of your cardiovascular and respiratory systems
- Efficiency of your metabolism
- Neuromuscular coordination

Sound familiar?

Some of this is your running biomechanics. Good running form is economical form. Wasted motion wastes energy. If you watched my video on running form on page 28, you know that I think you shouldn't change a thing if you are comfortable running and you're not getting injured. But I do like to see a midfoot strike because it keeps your foot underneath you when you land, which helps reduce the stress to your legs. A midfoot strike also means shorter ground-contact time. If you are a heel-striker, your foot hits the ground out in front of you, your leg is straighter, and there is more of a braking action going on (subtract energy points); and with your foot out in front, it forces you to pull your body forward (subtract more energy points) rather than push off the ground. To get a midfoot strike,

shorten your stride and increase your cadence: As you run, count every time your feet hit the ground for a minute. Your goal is 170 to 180 hits per minute. Also, think about your arms—not a lot; don't waste energy on worrying about your form—but ideally your arms are relaxed and moving forward and backward, not side to side across your body. When it comes to stability, the IronStrength workout will take care of that. Strong hips, glutes, and core will stop any rocking of the hips and wobbling at the knees and keep all of you pointed straight ahead.

Your vertical oscillation, or up-and-down displacement, will settle down to an efficient 5 to 7 centimeters simply by running. Here's the beautiful thing about your body: It wants to be efficient. It wants to conserve energy because it never knows when it is really going to need it—like when you're being chased by a saber-toothed tiger, right? And it wants to learn and improve at the activities that you love to do. So if you love running and you run regularly, your body will build a bigger, stronger heart; boost lung

MYTH BUSTER: LACTATE

. . . is not a waste product of metabolism.

. . . does not cause the burn you feel during intense running or any exercise.

. . . is not responsible for delayed-onset muscle soreness.

. . . does not cause fatigue.

capacity; improve neuromuscular coordination; make more mitochondria in your muscles; and become better at oxygen uptake and download, lactate shuttling, and all of the metabolic steps that go into producing the energy your muscles need to do the job.

Just as I mentioned earlier when talking about how to boost your body's ability to move and use oxygen, if you are a beginner, you will achieve leaps and bounds in running economy simply by running longer distances. In time, when your body has mastered the pace and distance you have set for it, you will need to up the challenge if you want to run faster. Here are the three best ways to strengthen your running economy for faster times.

1. **Speedwork.** If you think about all those physiological factors that influence how well you run—your ability to use oxygen, your lactate threshold, your running economy— what workout do you think does the best job of improving each and every one of those athletic attributes? Fast running. If you had to pick one type of training to help make you a better runner, this would be it. Training at a fast pace improves economy because your body makes the necessary adaptations in form and function to meet the requirements of that pace. Your body will make adjustments to deliver oxygen and move lactate more efficiently. It will create more mitochondria and build more capillaries. Your nerves and muscles will learn to work more efficiently for the neuromuscular coordination you need at a faster pace. And your body even learns that it shouldn't spend energy going up in the air when your goal is moving fast forward, so your vertical oscillation drops to an economical level. Your body improves its running economy to meet the demands of the pace that you run. So if your goal is to run your best 5-K, you need to include training at 5-K pace and faster in your schedule.

2. **Plyometrics.** When you think of muscle contraction, you usually think about the muscle shortening, right? Your biceps contract and shorten to lift your forearm, and this is called concentric muscle contraction. But there's another kind of muscle contraction that tends to cause muscle contortions in the faces of my patients when I talk about it—it's *eccentric* contraction. This occurs when your muscle lengthens as it contracts to resist force. (Yeah, I feel your pain.) The easiest example is the biceps curl: Your biceps contract and shorten as you lift the dumbbell, but as you lower it, your biceps lengthen at the same time that they contract to control the lowering of the weight. Let's look at your legs during running. As you swing your leg forward your calves and hamstrings lengthen, but just before your foot

hits the ground, they contract in preparation for landing and continue to contract to help control landing; then they push off with a concentric contraction. Confusing? A little. Brilliant? Big time. Because in that eccentric-to-concentric contraction, energy is quickly stored and used in push-off, and you spend less time on the ground (add points for economy). Plyometric strength training mimics the eccentric and concentric contractions of running, teaching you to be more efficient at them. I love efficiency, so it was a no-brainer to put plenty of plyometrics in my IronStrength program—building strength and economy into one workout.

3. **Hill training.** In my IronStrength classes in New York City, we begin the workout with some sprints up a hill. It's really hard, but I love to have runners do it because it builds a lot of strength in the legs and butt using real running movement. It's also really intense, so it will improve your lactate threshold and max VO_2. It gets you breathing hard. Your heart squeezes harder to pump more blood, and you become more efficient at extracting oxygen from your blood. This intense training over time improves your lactate threshold, meaning your fatigue level decreases the more you train.

Running hills is also a great way to improve your running economy. Hills force you to shorten your stride and use a midfoot strike. And they give your leg muscles lots of practice at eccentric contractions. On the way up the hill, your

DO YOU HIIT?

If you have ever trained at any level to improve your speed for racing, you have done it. HIIT is short for high-intensity interval training—short, intense bursts of exercise followed by equally short recoveries. It's the hottest thing to hit the exercise and fitness circuit since barefoot running. But we runners have known about it for years. The benefits are huge: Because of the high intensity and high demand for energy, it boosts oxygen intake, speeds metabolism, and dramatically increases your fitness. HIIT helps control blood insulin levels and improve insulin sensitivity, and it produces an afterburn effect that research has shown can burn calories for up to 24 hours postexercise.

If you are a seasoned competitive runner, you will customize HIIT to meet your training goals. For those of you who are new to running or who have been running for a while but never done intervals, here's how to give it a try: Warm up with 5 to 10 minutes of relaxed running, then run fast—not all out, but fast—for 60 seconds, recover for 2 minutes, and repeat three more times; finish up with some easy running. If 60 seconds of fast running seems hard (because it is), run 30 seconds fast and recover for 1 minute.

Start with just one HIIT workout a week. After about 4 weeks, you can add a second. I promise this workout will make you faster and make running more enjoyable. Go HIIT the road!

foot flexes upward more than if you were running on a flat surface, so your calves and Achilles tendons are stretched farther before your foot strikes the ground and your calves contract. On the way down, your quads get lots of practice with eccentric contractions, lengthening as you reach your leg forward and then quickly contracting to control knee motion as you land. Your hammys and calves also get a little more eccentric work since they have to elongate a little farther as you run downhill and contract a little harder to fight gravity at footstrike. Finally, you use your arms more when you run uphill and will naturally bring them into a forward-backward swing close to your body.

The best recipe for improved economy is some easy distance, some intense running (hills and intervals), and a little plyometrics—the same ingredients of a good training plan.

PUTTING IT ALL TOGETHER

We have covered a lot of ground here: the rules of healthy training, the physiology of running, and ways to make your physiology work harder for you. Now let's build a great plan that gets you to your running goals. I'm going to lay out all the different types of training and their effects and explain the proper paces for each type, and then we will look at how to arrange them in a sample training week.

Training Pieces

Different types of training produce different results, and the best plan links a variety of workouts so you can work on a few different skills at the same time. Here are all the different pieces to choose from to build your best training plan.

The long run. LSD—long, slow distance. The longest run of your week. This run builds your endurance and improves fat burning. Keep it easy. The running should be really comfortable, although you might begin to feel a little wobbly and achy during the last mile or two with all those steps under your feet.

Talk test: You should be able to have a conversation easily with a running buddy, no gasping for breaths between sentences.

The recovery run. Yep, just like the name implies, this is the run during which you recover from your previous day's run. If that seems confusing, think back to the principle of dynamic rest that I introduced in Chapter 1. You are continuing to exercise, but in a way that doesn't put strain on muscles that you pounded previously. You might choose to do a short, super-easy run or cross-train instead with some cycling or swimming.

Talk test: Your effort is so comfortable you could recite Shakespeare.

The plain-vanilla training run. This is when you're just heading out for a middle-of-the-road run (but of course, not *in* the middle of the road). It's not short or long, fast or slow, but it should still be comfortable like your long runs—before you've run your legs into the ground. What's the point? Practice, and learning to listen to your body, because you will let your body set the pace on these runs. Leave all training gadgets on the kitchen counter. Hit the road and go with the flow—run how you feel, faster on the days that you're stronger, slower on the days when your body is more tired. Just go and have fun. Sometimes plain vanilla tastes the best.

Talk test: You could hold a conversation easily or with a little bit of effort, depending on the pace your body picks.

The tempo run. This workout begins with a 10-minute warmup of easy running, then you shift into lactate threshold pace (85 percent of your mile pace) for 30 minutes, then ease back down and cruise to the finish. The tempo pace will be hard. If you have run a 10-K recently, it will be close to that pace. Tempo runs teach your body to adapt to the effort at which lactate starts piling up in your blood.

Talk test: You could spit out a few words here and there if you were willing to give up the oxygen.

Intervals. Now the effort skyrockets.

These workouts make you work really hard, but they also work really hard for you. Approach with caution, meaning warm up with a mile or two of running. Then you will do a series of short, fast runs, which could be anywhere from 100 meters to a mile in length, depending on your goal. How fast? At 90 to 100 percent of your 1-mile pace. In between the fast segments, you jog an easy recovery of the same or shorter distance. Interval training boosts your oxygen efficiency, raises your lactate threshold, and hones your running economy. Just do it.

Talk test: You won't be able to say a word.

Hills. There are a couple ways to approach hill training. You can choose to run hilly roads, which is a great choice for new runners or those who are just starting to add some harder workouts to their schedules. Or if you want a challenge, you can do hill repeats, which is essentially interval training on an incline. Here's how it works: Run a couple of easy miles to a hill that's at least 100 meters long, where you will sprint up, jog down, sprint up, jog down, etc. The steepness of the hill, the distance of the sprints, and the number of hill repeats you do depend on your training goal.

Talk test: As you run a rolling course you should be able to chat on the downhills, but you will be working too hard on the uphills to say anything. And hill repeats? Just lots of heavy breathing.

233

Training Paces

How fast is fast? How slow is slow? Time spent training will teach you your paces; you will learn what different efforts feel like. My friend Budd Coates describes in his book *Running on Air* a pacing method that relies on your attention to the rhythm of your breathing. What I love about Budd's strategy is that it emphasizes the mind–body connection, which can be so important not only to pacing during training and racing but also to injury prevention.

If you are someone who likes to run with a heart rate monitor, use these training zones:

- Recovery runs: 65 to 70 percent of max heart rate

Jen Darnell: The Running Scientist

I ran cross-country with the boys in high school because there was no girls' team. This was the late '70s in Indiana, and, on the track, girls were only allowed to run a mile—any longer was considered too strenuous. So I ran the mile. The only race time I remember was a 5:21 at regional championships during my sophomore year. Today, 36 years later, at age 52, I am a rejuvenated marathoner. I ran the New York City Marathon in 2010, finishing in 3 hours, 50 minutes and 28 seconds. Over the next 4 years, I dropped my time to 3 hours, 28 minutes and 8 seconds in the 2014 Boston Marathon, and I'm looking to finish my next marathon [Boston again, in 2015] even faster.

I am fortunate to have good genes—my max VO2 is very high—but the rest of it hasn't come easy. Though I ran competitively after college, I was stopped dead in my tracks in my late twenties by the blessing of four babies in 7 years, and I didn't begin running again until I turned 40. I started out on the elliptical and worked my way back to running on the roads. Eventually I decided I wanted to race again.

As I was training for the New York City Marathon, I developed iliotibial band syndrome, which led me to Dr. Metzl's office. I came away from that meeting with so much more than a prescription for healing. Dr. Metzl introduced me to IronStrength as well as several staff members at the Hospital for Special Surgery whom I have worked with over the past 4 years to fine-tune my training. For example, physiologist Polly de Mille ran some tests and discovered that I was burning too much glycogen—almost 100 percent even at a very slow pace. So I lowered my carb intake and now use 50 percent stored fat to fuel my marathons.

I also work with a trainer, a physical therapist, and a nutritionist at the hospital; became involved in the New York Athletic Club team; and found a coach, Greg McMillan, who understands my strengths and weaknesses. Working with all these experts and experimenting with my training have been

- Long runs and other easy runs: 75 to 85 percent of max heart rate
- Tempo runs and lactate threshold training: 88 to 92 percent of max heart rate
- Intervals: 95 to 100 percent

If you would rather not run with gadgetry, Budd offers an alternative: You can calculate your paces for different workouts from your fastest mile time. Your mile time sets the bar for your hardest training effort. It represents 100 percent. With that in mind, here's how your training efforts and paces break down.

Easy Runs/Long Runs

60 percent of mile pace

---

so valuable. I have learned that what works for me is to focus on quality training. I never run more than 55 miles a week, which includes one long run, one interval workout, and one tempo run. I use my foam roller almost every day, and thanks to plyometrics and strength training, I finally have glutes!

I recognize most runners don't have access to the kind of personal support group I'm so fortunate to have, but the strategy I have followed can help any runner improve. Two words define that strategy: education and experimentation. It's an approach I learned from my parents, who are both scientists, and from my career in scientific research as an associate professor of molecular neu-

roscience at The Rockefeller University.

First, learn as much as you can. Become a student of running. Read books and online articles by experts in training, nutrition, physiology, and sports medicine. Join a local team or running club, and cull from their experience.

Second, and equally important, experiment. No one understands your body and your life better than you. Keep a scientist's notebook, starting with the date and a title for the day's workout, and log all the data you can think of—details of your workout and of the life it's embedded in. Then experiment: Change one variable at a time and see what happens. You will have to repeat the experiment a

few times to see if it's reproducible. If you think you have discovered a pattern that helps or hinders your running, you might be able to devise an experiment to test whether you are right. Record the results and your conclusions in your notebook, and over time read back through your notes and analyze them for trends.

Finally, take all you have learned from the experts and from your own experiments and share it. Teaching others and inspiring them or helping them overcome the same roadblocks you have encountered is the biggest reward.

Tempo Runs/Lactate Threshold Training
85 percent of mile pace

Intervals
90 to 100 percent of mile pace
(depending on the workout)

When was the last time you raced a mile? If you are like me, never. Even if you *have* raced one, unless it was within the past month, you probably need to get your current time. Find a track or a flat road and time yourself running a mile as hard as you can. It would be really helpful if a running buddy would do this with you to help motivate you to your best effort. That mile represents your fastest training pace—100 percent. Your other training paces are calculated from there.

Let's say your best mile pace is 7 minutes.

100 percent effort is 7:00 per mile pace.
95 percent effort is 7:21 per mile pace.

The math:
7 minutes = 420 seconds
The difference in effort is 5 percent.
5 percent of 420 seconds = 21 seconds
A pace that is 5 percent *slower* than 7 minutes is 7:21.

Practice problem:
Your mile pace is 7 minutes. What would be your pace at an 85 percent effort?

7 minutes = 420 seconds
The difference in effort from 100 percent to 85 percent is _____ percent.

_____ percent of 420 seconds = _____ seconds

7 minutes + _____ seconds = _____

Your training paces based on a 7-minute mile would be as follows.

Intervals
90 to 100 percent: 7:42 to 7:00 per mile

Tempo runs/lactate threshold training
85 percent: 8:03 per mile

Easy runs/long runs
60 percent: 9:48 per mile

Training Schedules

You've got the pieces, you've got the paces. Next up—plugging different workouts into your training schedule using the following guidelines:

1. Follow a hard day of training with an easy day.

2. Increase your total weekly mileage by 10 percent. Remember, this is only a guide. Listen to your body and cut back if this increase feels like too much too soon. On the other hand, a highly experienced runner may be able to handle a slightly bigger increase.

3. Do not do more than two quality workouts—long run, intervals, tempo run, or hills—a week.

4. And don't go from zero to two hard runs in a week all at once. Add a hard workout and stay with it for about a month before adding the next hard run.

5. Over time, you will increase your weekly total mileage to a desired level based on your fitness, your goal, and how you choose to balance running with the rest of your life. But just as you plan recovery days into your week, it's a good idea to plan recovery weeks into your overall training, reducing mileage just a bit every other week before you jump to a higher level of mileage or intensity. For example, you might run 25 miles one week, increase to 27 the next week, and drop back to 25 before hitting 30 miles.

6. Training is usually developed around race goals. Once you have reached your goal, give your body a break and back off to a base level of comfortable training for a period before tackling the next big accomplishment on your running bucket list.

Remember to schedule in your Iron-Strength workout(s), and plan to exercise every day, even when you're not running.

Beginners. If you are brand-new to running, hopefully you've hung on through most of this chapter, because while some of the training detail might not be immediately relevant, all the information about physiology and its relationship to training does apply to you as you approach running and are trying to understand how to make this a healthy and enjoyable part of your life.

Start with 30 minutes, alternating walking and running, and do that four times a week. Keep in mind the hard/easy rule. Each week shorten the walking segments and increase your running time until you are running continuously for 30 minutes at a time.

SAMPLE WEEK	
Sunday	30-minute walk/run
Monday	cross-train (swim, bike, or yoga)
Tuesday	30-minute walk/run
Wednesday	30-minute walk/run
Thursday	IronStrength workout
Friday	30-minute walk/run
Saturday	cross-train (swim, bike, or yoga)

Fitness-and-Fun Runners. You're someone who loves to run but racing isn't really your thing. You run to maintain your health and weight, and you are so happy to go out for a plain-vanilla run with some friends—camaraderie at a comfortable pace. Here's a sample schedule for a 24- to 26-mile week.

SAMPLE WEEK	
Sunday	6 to 8 miles
Monday	cross-train (swim, bike, or yoga)
Tuesday	5 miles
Wednesday	5 miles
Thursday	IronStrength workout
Friday	5 miles
Saturday	cross-train (swim, bike, or yoga)

I like you to have one run that's a little longer each week to build a little more endurance. Endurance is a good thing, and a long run is an accomplishment. It makes you feel like you've got some mojo, and it will help you step to higher mileage or more intense training if you decide you want a new challenge. I'm not saying you ever have to do any more than a set amount of miles a week, because you don't. But know that your body adapts, and if you want to see gains in fitness, you will need to add some intensity or distance, or both. A simple way to add some intensity to your week is by taking a little HIIT of it (check out "Do You HIIT?" on page 231).

Competitive Runners. You love racing against yourself and other runners, hunting down your rivals on the course or going for a PR. And the rush when you get one, when you push over the finish line under the race clock and under your previous best—victory is sweet! To get there you have to build a training plan with all the pieces: long runs, intervals, hills, tempo runs, strength training, and rest. You have to train smart. If you dump all that intense training into every week, you will be fast, all right—fast on the way to injury, and you can kiss your race goals goodbye. Add hard workouts the way you do mileage—gradually. Start with one high-intensity workout a week for a month or so before adding a second. And pay attention to pain; adding speed workouts is a lot harder

on your body than adding miles. If you have discomfort that alters the way you run, you need to stop and figure out what's going on. If you feel that you're overtraining—you are fatigued, grumpy, and your speed workouts are subpar—cut back on your mileage or intensity or both until you feel recovered and ready for more.

SAMPLE WEEK	
Sunday	long run
Monday	easy run or cross-train (swim, bike, or yoga)
Tuesday	moderate run
Wednesday	hard workout (intervals, tempo, or hills)
Thursday	IronStrength
Friday	moderate run
Saturday	day off, easy run, or cross-train (swim, bike, or yoga)

Building a training schedule for racing is complicated. How you put the pieces together depends on your level of fitness, the level of commitment you are able to give to training, your race goal, and the philosophy of training that you feel comfortable with and that you believe will bring you success. There is no one exact best way to train for any race, and there are many great training programs available. Choose a plan and stay with it for a couple of years; then consider trying a different approach to training. Changing things up challenges your body in new ways to build even better running and racing fitness.

CHAPTER 14

UNLEASH YOUR BIGGEST WEAPON

Silent (mostly) but powerful, the brain controls it all. Nothing happens without a command from the gray matter, whether you will it to happen—like getting up from the chair you're sitting in—or the action is on permanent autopilot, like the beating of your heart.

Your brain directs all of your physiology, and as you run that means muscle contractions, heartbeats, breathing, bloodflow, metabolism, and neuromuscular coordination. You become a better runner through training because your brain learns that to perform at a higher level, all this stuff has to happen: You need stronger leg muscles, a stronger heart, more powerful lungs, a more efficient form, a more efficient metabolism. And your brain sends out signals to the players in your physiology that they need to build muscle, create more mitochondria in your cells for energy production, produce more enzymes for metabolism, and on and on. The speed and synchronicity of nerve signals and physiological responses that produce the movement that propels you down the road is remarkable.

Then there are the intangibles of your mind—emotions, stress, psychological energy, and mental fatigue. These impact your performance too. We can't measure them directly; I have yet to come across a stress-o-meter or a gauge to measure how happy you are. We measure stress, happiness, fear, anger, calm by looking at physiological responses, so clearly our thoughts and emotions have an impact on our bodies. And though it often seems that what's going on inside your head has a mind of its own, you get to call the shots—quiet the trash talk and raise the volume on positive, constructive thinking—in ways that benefit your metabolic efficiency and your running economy.

TO LISTEN OR NOT TO LISTEN? THAT IS THE QUESTION

Which of these two camps are you in?

1. When I'm running or racing, I like to listen to music or try to think about things that take my mind off any discomfort I feel. If I paid attention to the effort I was putting out or how many more miles I had to run, I would probably just stop.

2. I don't listen to anything when I run. I want to feel the "slings and arrows," which are the essence of running. When I'm alone with my thoughts, my brain works wonders. I also find that I can focus on pace and concentrate on keeping my form intact.

If you are in the first camp, you like to *dissociate* from your body when you run.

If you are in the second camp, you prefer to *associate* with your running body.

What's the best camp to be in? How about both?

Since I'm a sports doctor, I am always paying attention to what's going on with my body during a race. I evaluate every little ache and pain. And—

since I'm a sports doctor—I know right away whether that ache or pain is something I can run with or something that might blow up into an injury. As an experienced competitive athlete, I know that it's going to hurt to race my best. I have also learned how to sustain a pace at some level of pain. Discomfort does not deep-six my performance, and it doesn't have to deep-six yours.

If you focus on fatigue and the strain of hard running or you worry too much about how well you will perform, it will mess with your head, making you fearful or anxious—and that mental tension creates physical tension. Your heart rate goes up, your breathing rate increases, and energy is produced that doesn't reach your running muscles because it gets gobbled up by clenched muscles (it's work to clench your muscles). In other words, you're throwing energy away on anxiety, energy that could be conserved and used to fuel running.

You need to find a way to clear your mind of toxic thoughts and emotions, but you still need to keep your head in the game if you want to run your best. Dissociation is fine for an easy or moderate run, with these two caveats.

1. Never ignore pain that changes the way you run! I can't emphasize enough how bad injuries are made into really bad injuries by running through pain that is changing the mechanics of how you are running.

2. If your easy run is a recovery run, stay at a recovery pace.

In a race, however, focus gets you to the finish line faster. You need to tune in to your body to fine-tune your performance. Don't just look at the mile clocks to determine if you are on the right pace. Check in with your physical status. How hard are you breathing? How do your legs feel? Can you push a little harder or should you back off a hair? What's up with your upper

SILENCE PRERACE ANXIETY

Back in 2005, I raced the Ironman World Championship triathlon in Hawaii. I prepared really well, but as the race approached, I felt increasingly excited but also nervous and agitated. Questions raced through my brain: Will a shark see me as his next meal? Will the infamous winds of Kona topple my bike? Will I bonk before I reach the finish line? Worry is nothing more than wasted energy—literally. Anxiety creates physiological expenditures in the form of rapid breathing, increased heart rate, and sweating. Your sleep may get disrupted, which only elevates

anxiety (please don't worry if you don't sleep the night before a race, though; it will not affect your performance, I promise). So what should you do when prerace jitters jostle your confidence? You need to quiet the voices and find your calm. I use visualization.

In the days before a big event, I picture myself running strong and smooth, in good form, with controlled breathing and a smile on my face. By steering my mind to positive visions of perfect performance, fear and anxiety disappear.

body? (Shoulders tend to tense up toward the end of a race.)

Don't expect to show up on race day and know how to funnel your mental energy away from discomfort, doubt, and fear and into finessing your run-ning. You train your muscles for per-formance; you need to train your mind too. The strategies are simple, and not only will they benefit your race times, but they will also enhance your entire running experience too.

DISCONNECT TO CONNECT

I like yoga because it gives you a little more physical flexibility. It's especially good for endurance athletes who ham-mer their muscles on the road for a long, long time. But the benefits stretch even further: Yoga trains your mind for three important skills.

- How to relax mind and muscle
- How to clear your head of self-doubt, anxiety, and fear
- How to focus your mental energy

The Art of Breathing

Central to the practice of yoga is the art of breathing. Though we take it for granted because we do it constantly without thinking, breathing can be a powerful force for good in your run-ning world. You can use it to clear your mind, find your calm, and con-nect mind and body. By focusing on your breathing, you pull your mind away from the clamor of negative thinking: "This is too hard." "It hurts too much." "I can't keep up this pace." "Oh man, look at that hill." "What, I've got 3 miles to go? I'll never make it."

Breathe. Let your mind follow the air in and out, in and out. As you focus on your breathing, the noise in your head will quiet down and you will relax. Some people find it helpful to create a mantra and repeat it each time they exhale. Say to yourself, "Relax, relax, relax." And imagine that with every exhale you are pushing anxiety, self-doubt, and discomfort right out of your body. Your mind relaxes, your body follows, and as you calm down your running performance rises up.

BREATHE THIS WAY

Breathing to relax mind and body should be deep, using your diaphragm to fully expand your lungs. Focus on breathing from your belly instead of your chest, where breaths will be shallow. To check your breathing style, lie down and place your hand on your abdomen; it should rise and fall as you breathe. If it's not, focus on breathing from your belly. Prac-tice until it comes naturally.

10 WAYS RUNNING BOOSTS YOUR BRAIN

I exercise for a lot of reasons, but some of the most important are the ways it benefits my brain. Exercise gives me more mental energy and sharpens my focus and thinking so I can be at my best with every patient I see during the day—and I see a lot of patients. Here are 10 ways running can make a difference in the health of your mind.

1. Relieve stress
2. Induce relaxation
3. Lift depression
4. Crank up mental energy
5. Expand creativity
6. Improve learning, memory, and cognitive skills
7. Sharpen focus
8. Boost self-esteem
9. Make you feel in control
10. Grow new brain cells

The Center of Your Mental Energy Universe

Centering is a common practice in yoga, meditation, and martial arts and can have a big payoff for running too. Imagine a point in your body at or below your navel—that's your center. As you breathe, exhale away all the negative junk that's been filling your head and then redirect your energy to your center. Think of it as a place of calm and stability inside you. Remember how I talked about the importance of physical stability in your hips and how that helps keep your body aligned and prevents wasted motion? Centering is the mental equivalent. When you are centered, you don't get rattled by worries about your performance. You have a quiet inner strength that nothing can shake and from which you can comfortably control your performance.

The Mind–Body Connection

Once you have stopped listening to negative voices, pushed away anxiety, and settled into a relaxed and centered mind-set, you are ready to use your mind to power your performance. And you do that through focused attention on your body and its movement.

You hear coaches all the time tell their athletes to listen to their bodies, and for good reason: Your body can tell you what's going on, like "We know that adrenaline encouraged you to shoot off the starting line like a rocket, but we need to back off and settle into race pace, please." How do you interpret what your body is trying to say? Pay attention in training. Breathing is an excellent gauge of effort—run harder and faster and you breathe deeper and quicker; run slower and breathing slows and becomes more comfortable. Because oxygen is directly connected to energy production and effort, breathing is an immediate response to effort and pace. Focus on it when you run easy, when you run uphill, when you run intervals. Over time you will learn what different efforts, aka paces, feel like. You will be

243

able to check in with your breathing to find out whether you are running too fast, too slow, or just right. Keeping the right running pace is a pretty significant factor in finishing a 5-mile run or a 5-mile race.

You also want to work your mind–body connection to improve your running economy. By taking an inventory of your body from head to toe while you run, you can identify glitches and correct them. If a muscle feels tense, use your relaxation skills to release it. A pain in your leg might be resolved by changing your cadence for several yards. Evaluate your arm swing, and if you notice too much side-to-side motion, gently bring your arms back to a forward-backward swing. Shoulders tend to get tense toward the end of a long run or race; if you feel tightness there, shake your arms out at your sides and then get back to the road ahead. By checking in with your body regularly during a race and making any minor corrections, running will become more comfortable, and you can shave precious seconds off your finish time.

Picture This

In the days leading up to a big race, I play the event in my mind like a movie. I see it all from beginning to end, and everything goes just right. Before a triathlon, I imagine swimming smoothly, streamlined, gliding through the water with tropical fish at my side. I see myself cruising down the road on my bike with the wind at my back. And finally, the run: arms swinging comfortably at my side, my steps light, my stride strong. I am pain-free and smiling.

Sports psychologists call this visualization. I like to call it your mental dress rehearsal. You know that mind–body connection you are going to work on? Visualization is your mind's way of taking your body through its paces without you actually having to run them. (How great is that?) It helps

---

PUT PAIN IN ITS PLACE

Discomfort can do a real number on your head. It makes you think you need to slow down or, worse, stop altogether. And sometimes that's true. Explosive, acute injuries—an ankle sprain, a tear to a tendon—will stop you in your tracks. But achy pain or soreness doesn't have to pull you over to the side of the road, unless it causes you to change your form or run differently than you would normally. In that case, you do want to call it quits because continuing will make the injury worse and may create an additional problem.

If the discomfort you're feeling is the pain that comes with physical exertion, try to reframe it. Dissociate from it; see it as something separate from you. Use it as a tool to gauge your effort. When you can objectify pain, you take away its power, and then *you're* in control.

alleviate prerace anxiety, and it is the ultimate application of the power of positive thinking—think it and it will happen. Of course, I'm not suggesting that you can think yourself onto the Olympic team, but you can certainly think yourself to better performance.

On race day, you can play another kind of mind game. Answer this: If as a runner you could be a smooth, quick animal or some flowing force of nature, like a stream, what would you be? A cheetah? A gazelle? The wind? As you run, see yourself as the cheetah, the flowing water. The imagination is powerful. Whatever image you choose will inspire your confidence. Picturing fast, fluid movement motivates your own speed and efficiency, and it can be a terrific tool to help banish evil thinking and center your mind on the positive. If you are someone who never steps foot on the starting line of a race, it's still really great to imagine yourself as a gazelle.

Running Is a Journey, Not a Destination

It's great to have goals, right? I love goals, and I set race goals every single year. It's something to go after, something to get excited about, something to keep me motivated. And then there's achieving the goal or even surpassing it. What a rush it was for me to have raced a PR in my 12th Ironman triathlon at Lake Placid.

One of the great things about our sport is that you can improve at any level, and that improvement is self-

affirming. It builds confidence. But if a goal becomes your entire focus, it will consume you. If the need to beat your fiercest competitor, to get that next PR, or to qualify for the Boston Marathon becomes too entwined with your feelings of self-worth, the good medicine of running goes bad. When the desire to win—however you define it personally—becomes too intoxicating, your judgment becomes clouded. You might not make the best decisions about how to get to your goal. You might ignore a brewing injury or succumb to overtraining. The end result is that you don't achieve your dream and you suffer trying to get there. It hurts physically, and it hurts emotionally.

When you set your eyes on the prize alone, you lose sight of what's right in front of you, which is the run you are taking today, whether an easy 3 miles or 3 miles of hill repeats. Focus on today's run, today's goal, and do it to the best of your ability—that's how you become a better runner, the best runner you can be. That's how you will reach your goals; no other way will get you there better or faster. That's how you will stay healthy physically and mentally, and how running contributes to your best life.

Brain Training

You might be wondering if all these mental strategies—relaxation, centering, visualization—really work or if it's all a lot of hooey. It's a fair question. After all, how, for example, do scientists measure centering in the laboratory? What researchers can measure is running performance among individuals who practice these techniques against those who don't. And what studies indicate is that runners who use relaxation techniques to eliminate negative thinking and emotion, practice centering, visualize performance, and focus on what they need to do to train for their best race improve their running economy and consequently their performance.

But again, these aren't tricks to pull out of your singlet at the starting line. By practicing these skills in training, they will become your go-to mental strategies on race day. Where to fit mind work into your running schedule? You can practice it every time you go for a run, but since these skills will help you take command of the race course, you definitely want to use them on your hard days: long runs, tempo runs, hill runs, and intervals—the workouts that test you physically and mentally.

I love these strategies for strengthening your mind and your mind–body connection, but know too that *all* training builds a powerful brain. Long runs, hills, and intervals take both body and brain through the hard work. As I pointed out at the beginning of this chapter, your brain is the real mastermind. It controls muscular contractions, muscle-fiber recruitment, metabolism, enzyme production, and so much more. And your brain's number-one job is to protect the organism. Physical effort is a threat. It uses energy, oxygen, and water; it strains your musculoskeletal system; and it raises the temperature of your body. Your brain will go conservative on you if it doesn't know what you can handle.

Running hard teaches your brain what it needs to do under difficult physiological situations. Your brain learns what you are capable of and how to respond. So when you come up to a hill on a training run or in a race, your brain knows you can do this because you have done it before, and it delivers what your body needs—no hesitation, no questions asked.

Your brain is like the conductor of a symphony orchestra. Give her the score for the first time and no matter how talented the musicians or how well they know the piece, that first performance will be just okay. As the conductor and orchestra practice together over and over again, the conductor learns what's required of the music and gets to know the capabilities of the musicians, and that's when she directs a standing ovation–worthy performance.

PART IV

Tools of the Trade

Tools? What tools? One of the reasons we love running is because it is so unencumbered. Good food. Good shoes. A long road. And you're on your way. Well, yes, you *will* need to put on some clothes, too, before you step out the door.

CHAPTER 15

GOOD FOOD

Do you eat to run or do you run to eat? If you answered the latter, you have lots of friends—including me. The joy of running for me is also the joy of being able to eat.

I love to eat. I love food. I'm a pizza-holic, and I love a good hamburger more than the next guy. And I love dessert. But I also love being healthy, so I eat a lot of healthy foods too. And I listen to my body in all things, including the way my diet makes me feel. I'm tuned in, and I know when I'm all sugared up or when I'm a little heavier or feeling lethargic, and I will make changes as I need to.

So you can see I'm not an absolutist. I haven't banned any food from my diet. But I am a realist. And the truth is

there are good carbs and there are not-so-good carbs; good fats and not-so-good fats; good proteins and not-so-good proteins. And while you may be one of those runners who can eat anything and everything and not gain a pound, that doesn't mean what you put in your mouth won't affect what you put out in performance on the road or the quality of your health now and later. You wear the best shoes for running health and performance, right? Why not eat the best foods too? It matters. Let me tell you why.

THE FOODS WE HATE TO LOVE

Unfortunately, the least healthy calories are found in some of our most favorite foods.

Sugar—Not So Sweet

Got a sweet tooth? Think before you bite into that second doughnut or grab another handful of malted milk balls or pour yourself a 32-ounce ginger ale at the soda fountain. Yummy? Yes. Good for you? Maybe if you're in the middle of a marathon and you have used up all your glycogen stores, but in your daily diet? No.

One of the biggest reasons nutritionists don't want you eating lots of cookies, candy, and other sweets is that they take up caloric space that could be given to nutrient-rich foods, like fruits, vegetables, and whole grains. How much vitamin C does a glazed doughnut give you? Zero.

But sugar isn't just a benign consumer of your daily calories; it can do some serious damage to your health. Too much sugar messes with brain chemicals and has been linked to depression, learning problems, anxiety, and poor memory. It depresses your hormonal response to eating, short-circuiting the signals that tell you you're full, which isn't very helpful if you are trying to lose weight. Researchers have linked high sugar consumption to high blood pressure, increased blood fats, low HDL (good cholesterol), a fatty liver, stiff arteries, and even breast and colon cancer. In a study published in the January 2014 issue of *JAMA Internal Medicine*, scientists examined data from the National Health and

FOOD CHEMISTRY 101: CARBS EXPLAINED

Glucose is a simple sugar. When you eat carbohydrates—pasta, for example—your body breaks them down into glucose molecules, which are used to produce energy or are stored as glycogen in your muscles and liver.

Fructose is another simple sugar and is the type common in fruit. It is also added to soda and sweetened drinks. It is not metabolized in the same way that glucose is, so it gets sent to your liver.

Sucrose comes from sugarcane or sugar beets and is the table sugar you spoon into your coffee. Sucrose is a combination of fructose and glucose.

Starches are a lot of glucoses linked together in long chains; when you eat them, digestion breaks apart the chains into individual glucose molecules.

Refined carbohydrates include sugar and starches that have been stripped of fiber and most nutrients—foods like white pasta, white rice, white bread, and cereals such as Lucky Charms.

Complex carbohydrates have their fiber and nutrients intact. These include whole grains—such as brown rice and whole grain pasta, cereal, and breads—as well as all fruits and vegetables.

Nutrition Examination Survey, which collected information about diet habits from more than 30,000 US adults over a 15-year period. The researchers found that individuals who took in 17 to 21 percent of daily calories from added sugar had a 38 percent higher risk of dying from heart disease than those who consumed less than 10 percent, and that was regardless of sex, age, physical activity, and BMI. Seeing data like that, the American Heart Association recommends that women limit added sugar to 100 calories a day (25 grams, 6 teaspoons, 5 percent of a 2,000-calorie diet) and men stop at 150 calories daily (37.5 grams, 9 teaspoons, 7.5 percent of a 2,000-calorie diet). To get a taste of the high sugar content of some beloved sweet treats, take a look at these numbers.

CALORIES FROM SUGAR		
1	12-ounce can of soda	140 sugar calories
1	large blueberry muffin, about 3 inches in diameter	182 sugar calories
1	8-ounce (really small) chocolate milk shake	248 sugar calories

But I run and I need sugar to fuel my running, you say. I'm just going to burn it up, right? On a long run, a marathon, even a half-marathon, getting a quick sugar fix—say, from a sports beverage or gel—is a great idea. Your muscles will be thankful. They will suck it right up, and sugars won't

be roaming around your body causing disruption. But for day-to-day eating and training, complex carbohydrates are the way to go (more on that later).

Saturated Fat—A Big Fat No-No

Fat packs a lot of calories—9 for every gram versus 4 for every gram of carbohydrate or protein that you put in your mouth. But the real health hazard of saturated fat (emphasis on the word *saturated*) is that it raises LDL cholesterol, the evil cholesterol that can lead to heart disease and stroke. There has been some buzz over research showing that saturated fat is not linked to heart disease, but those were observational studies, which show an association between two facts, not cause and effect. The gold standard of research—controlled clinical studies—time and time again shows that a diet high in saturated fat produces high levels of LDL in the bloodstream, which in turn raises risk of cardiovascular disease.

The American Heart Association recommends we all limit our daily saturated fat consumption—butter, full-fat dairy products, high-fat meats—to 5 to 6 percent of total calories a day. For a 2,000-calorie diet, that comes to 120 calories, or 13 grams of fat. A typical single-patty cheeseburger packs 15 to 16 grams and puts the average person just over the top. Does that mean you must ban burgers at the backyard barbecue? Not at all. Just don't eat them every day, and when you do have one, be more vigilant about avoiding foods high in saturated fat the rest of the week.

Trans Fats—Your Greatest Foe

If you thought saturated fat was bad, check this out: Trans fats, or trans fatty acids, not only raise LDL cholesterol, but they also lower your HDLs (the good one). It's a double hit to your cardiovascular system. Bad stuff. In fact, in 2013 the US Food and Drug Administration decided to keep trans fats off their GRAS (generally recognized as safe) list. Trans fats are most common in packaged snacks, baked goods, and many fried foods. How much trans fat is okay to eat? Zero. Nada. Don't consume any of it. And when you see a food labeled no trans fat, know this: Food companies are allowed to make that claim if the amount of trans fat is below 0.5 gram. I'm not sure when a half a gram of anything equaled zero—sounds like funny math to me—but you can outsmart the companies that are trying to pull a fast one on you by checking the ingredients list of packaged foods. If you see partially hydrogenated oil of any kind, put that processed product right back on the grocery store shelf.

SUPERFOODS

These foods save the day every day by giving you energy to burn, rebuilding muscle and bone, and making you feel like a superhero.

Complex Carbohydrates

Your best source of energy, complex carbs deliver premium fuel for working muscles. This food group includes all whole grains as well as all fruits and vegetables. In your gut, these foods are broken down into glucose, which is transported throughout your body in your bloodstream. Some of that glucose is used immediately for energy production, but most is stored as glycogen in your muscles and in your liver for future use. The beautiful thing about complex carbs is that they have all their fiber on, which slows the release of glucose into your bloodstream. You don't get that crazy sugar rush and crash.

The other great thing about complex carbs is that they are loaded with vitamins and minerals that help with everything from regulating metabolism to building bone, blood, and muscle cells to boosting immune function and protecting you from disease, including cardiovascular diseases and cancer. This is the biggest food group of all. You have a huge variety to choose from—and lots to love: whole grain bread, oatmeal, corn, broccoli, asparagus, carrots, sweet potatoes, greens, squash, beets, cauliflower, strawberries, blueberries, blackberries, melons,

DO YOU NEED SUPPLEMENTS?

My philosophy is simple: By eating a wide variety of whole foods, you can get all the nutrients your body needs for optimal health and running performance. A supplement is exactly that—a supplement to what you're eating, not a replacement.

Certain situations, however, may call for supplementation. Women at high risk for osteoporosis—including those who are of northern European descent and/or have fair skin and blue eyes—may need to take calcium if they are not getting enough from their diets. Low-fat dairy products are the best source, but if you are vegan or just don't like dairy, you may fall short on your needs for this essential mineral.

Omega-3s are important to heart health, and many of us don't get enough. The best source is fatty fish. Try to eat two servings of fish a week along with plant sources, such as flaxseed and chia seeds. Not a fish lover? Then you should think about popping a few omega-3 supplements daily.

tomatoes, peaches, apples, pears, kiwifruit, mango, papaya, green beans, peas, and the list goes on and on and on and on. Eat the widest variety of fruits and veggies that you can. Plant foods not only deliver lots of vitamins and minerals but are also rich in antioxidants and phytochemicals that power up your health. Nutrition scientists are constantly discovering new health benefits in individual fruits and veggies, so your best strategy is to eat them all, and lots of them.

Lean Proteins

To build a super body, you need super building materials. Like the lumber used in your home, protein is the raw material your body needs for construction, and not just for making muscle. Protein is used to build and repair tendons and ligaments, construct new capillaries, produce the enzymes and mitochondria needed in metabolism, and strengthen your heart. A little bit is also burned for fuel. What's the best protein for all these jobs? The lean ones with the least amount of saturated fat: lean beef, pork, and poultry, as well as beans, lentils, soy foods, eggs, low-fat dairy products, and some veggies (all veggies have a gram or two of protein, but certain ones—like avocado—have a little more).

When serving up seafood, however, turn your fat meter off. The healthiest fishes are the fatty ones: salmon, mackerel, tuna (canned and fresh), lake trout, herring, and sardines. These contain omega-3 fatty acids—powerful polyunsaturated fatty acids that may help decrease triglycerides (bad fats in the blood), lower cholesterol and blood pressure, reduce inflammation throughout your body, and even make you smarter. Smart vegetarians will sprinkle some ground flaxseed or chia seeds in their cereals, salads, and stir-fries. Both are rich in omega-3s, and chia seeds deliver a decent amount of protein too.

Now, if you're vegetarian, getting all the protein you need will be a little more challenging for you than for your meat-eating friends, and tougher still if you are a vegan. Some of the best non-meat sources of protein include eggs (see "Humpty Dumpty" on page 258), lentils, beans, soy foods, Greek yogurt, low-fat dairy foods, quinoa, avocado (3 grams in a cup, plus all nine essential amino acids), nuts, and seeds. You do not need to eat complementary proteins together at the same meal as was once thought, but you do need to eat a variety of protein-rich foods—and plenty of them, since protein is not as readily absorbed from plant sources.

The same is true of iron. Red meat is the iron king. Popeye made it look easy, but this crucial mineral is not so easily absorbed from plant foods. Vitamin C enhances absorption though, so throw some red bell peppers into your stir-fry or orange slices into your spinach salad.

Then there's this little fun fact to consider: As you pound the pavement, you are literally crushing red blood cells. The farther you run, the more of these vital oxygen carriers you stomp out. To produce more red blood cells, your body needs iron to make hemoglobin, the protein in your red blood cells that holds oxygen. What does this all mean? If you are vegetarian, you may fall short of your iron needs. Make an extra effort to eat iron-rich foods, and pay attention to your iron intake and your energy levels. If you notice that you feel fatigued day after day and your running seems to slog along, see your doctor.

Monounsaturated Fats

We talked about how omega-3s are good for your health. Well, here's another class of fats that you want to consume: monounsaturated fats—the heroes of your heart. They lower LDL cholesterol while raising HDLs, and they improve your body's absorption of certain carotenoids from vegetables. (Carotenoids help reduce your risk of heart disease and certain cancers.)

Monounsaturated fats made big news in a study of the heart-protective effect of the Mediterranean diet. In this huge study involving more than 7,000 men and women at high risk for cardiovascular disease, researchers compared a low-fat diet to the Mediterranean diet. The two meal plans were not dissimilar—lots of fruits and vegetables and lean

SPREAD IT OUT

You could consume all the calcium you need in a day at breakfast with a calcium-fortified whole grain cereal drenched with calcium-rich milk plus a big glass of calcium-boosted orange juice to wash down your calcium supplement, but that's a poor plan. Your body can only absorb so much calcium at a time—500 milligrams being the max—so eat your high-calcium foods throughout the day.

VITAMIN SUPER-C

Vitamin C does amazing work for your body. An antioxidant, it helps prevent cell damage from free radicals—unstable molecules that are formed in various ways, including during metabolism, and which damage muscle cells and other healthy tissue by stealing electrons from molecules that make up that tissue. Vitamin C is also part of several building and repair crews. It is used to form a protein for building tendons and ligaments and for shoring up the walls of blood vessels. It helps repair and maintain cartilage and bones, and it boosts absorption of iron and folate. Lots of great reasons to enjoy plenty of high-C fruits and vegetables, such as the citruses, berries, greens, broccoli, red bell peppers, and more.

proteins. But the Mediterranean diet group had to consume 4 or more tablespoons of extra-virgin olive oil or 30 grams—a handful—of nuts high in monounsaturated fat every day. The result? The men and women who followed the Mediterranean diet lowered their risk of cardiovascular disease and death by a whopping 30 percent. The results were so amazing that the researchers cut the study short after 5 years so they could share their life-saving news with the rest of the world.

Olive oil is an excellent source of monounsaturated fats, but so are canola oil, nuts, olives, peanut butter and other nut butters, and avocados.

Low-Fat Dairy

Here's a good reason to wear a milk moustache—calcium. You already know that calcium builds strong bones, but how about these other important jobs? It plays a role in muscle contraction and the regulation of your heartbeat; it helps your nerves send messages and your blood vessels move blood; and it assists in the release of hormones and enzymes. Your body really puts this mineral to work, so you need to make sure you are replenishing your stores every day. Here are the daily recommended amounts, according to the National Institutes of Health.

YOUR DAILY CALCIUM	
Teens 14–18	1,300 milligrams
Adults 19–50	1,000 milligrams
Men 51–70	1,000 milligrams
Women 51–70	1,200 milligrams
Adults 71+	1,200 milligrams

Low-fat milk, yogurt, and cheese are rich in calcium that's easily absorbed by your body. But if you don't like dairy or are lactose intolerant or vegan, other good sources include kale; broccoli; Chinese cabbage; grains; and fortified cereals, juices, and soy products. Your body will have a much easier time absorbing calcium when vitamin D is around, which is why vitamin D is added to dairy and fortified foods.

EAT TO RUN: A RUNNER'S DAILY DIET

So how do all these different foods—the healthy and the not-so-healthy—play out on your plate? Let me start by saying this: Low-carb diets and endurance sports don't go hand in hand. Sports researchers have been cooking up some different ideas about eating for endurance. Some theorize that low-carb diets might teach your body to rely less on glucose and more on fat for fuel. Others have proposed that if you eat more fat, you will burn more fat. Interesting ideas for sure, but I haven't seen solid scientific evidence to support either. My advice? Stick with the tried-and-true general guidelines: 60 percent or more of your calories should come from carbohydrates, 15 to 20 percent from protein, and 20 to 25 percent from fat. The longer and harder you run, the more carbs and protein you should consume.

I also like—literally and philosophically—eating throughout the day: three meals with snacks in between. I eat all day long. Even though I see patients pretty much nonstop when I'm at work, I will steal a minute or two here and there to slip into my office and grab a handful of almonds or some dried fruit from my stash.

Aim for a mix of carbs, protein, and fats at each feeding. This strategy provides a slow and steady release of carbohydrates into your bloodstream so that those carbs get used as energy and stored as glycogen, not packed into fat cells. This also prevents a sugar high followed by an energy crash. Go for the good carbs—fruits and vegetables and whole grains—lean proteins, and mostly monounsaturated fats. Does this mean no burgers, no pizza, no dessert? Well, I would be a hypocrite if I told you never to eat any of those foods. And besides, when you deprive yourself of something you really enjoy, you are much more likely to gorge on it when you do get a taste. So go ahead and eat what you like, but in moderation. Fill up most of your plate with good-for-you foods.

And don't forget to drink all day long too (nonalcoholic beverages, of course). Many of us neglect to sip enough fluids during the day because our thirst mechanism isn't as strong as hunger, and it's easy to ignore it when we are busy. Try to get into the habit of having a water bottle with you and sipping regularly. If good old H_2O doesn't inspire you, purchase an infuser bottle and flavor your water with fruit. All nonalcoholic beverages, including coffee, count toward your fluid intake, as do water-laden whole fruits and veggies, which are a far better choice than juices with little fiber and loads of sugar. You don't have to do any math on your fluid intake every day, just check your urine: If it's pale, give yourself two thumbs up; medium to dark, drink more water.

Prerun and Postworkout

Assuming you eat regularly throughout the day, you likely won't need a prerun snack. But if you are a first-thing-in-the-morning runner, you need to replenish glycogen and fluids that were used up while you slept. Eat a high-carb, easily digested snack at least 30 minutes before you hit the road. Some yummy options: cereal with milk, yogurt and fruit, a bagel with cream cheese, a smoothie, or toast and a banana. And have some water with that.

If you're heading for a run of 2 hours or more, you might want to take some carbs with you in the form of sports gels or applesauce packets. These are best taken with water, so run a route that takes you past a water fountain or carry water with you. Keep in mind that training runs are the time and place to practice your race-day nutrition strategy. So if you think you might want to eat a sports bar before your race or take an energy gel or sports beverage during the race, try them out on a training run to learn how compatible they are with your digestive tract, as well as how effective they will be at fueling your running.

After your workout, you need to restock your glycogen stores and water reserves and start repairing muscle. Research has shown that a postwork-out snack that delivers carbs and protein in a ratio of 4-to-1 is the ideal. And what favorite childhood beverage has now become the go-to recovery drink? If you guessed chocolate milk, you are absolutely correct. (Yes! Permission to drink chocolate milk!) Don't like chocolate milk or can't drink it? Have a PB&J on whole grain bread; make a smoothie with yogurt, fruit, and a scoop of protein powder; or have yogurt with fruit and a sprinkling of nuts. And take a look at some of the sports nutrition bars for quick and easy post-workout replenishment. Sports nutritionists say you don't have to hit that 4-to-1 ratio of carbs to protein exactly, but they do recommend that you try to get 0.5 gram of carbs per pound of body weight. So if you weigh 150 pounds, that's 75 grams of carbohydrates, or 300 calories. Add 75 calories of protein (19 grams) and you're there. For optimal recovery after your workout, be sure to eat your postrun snack within 15 minutes of stopping.

And don't forget to replace the fluids you sweated out as you ran. (You will be pretty thirsty, so you're likely to remember.) If the heat and humidity are high and you ran for an hour or more, drink a sports beverage to replace electrolytes. To figure out how much fluid you need to replace after running, weigh yourself before your workout and then again when you're done, and drink 16 ounces for every pound you dropped.

EAT TO RACE: A RUNNER'S PREMIUM FUEL

Have I told you yet how much I love to eat and that I eat everything? However, a month before an important competition—a marathon or an Iron-man that I have been focused on—I will clean out my diet. I cut out simple sugars, fried foods, and fatty foods and focus on lots of veggies, lean proteins, and whole grain breads and pastas. And in the days right before the race, I carbo-load.

Runners have been carbo-loading for marathons since the '70s, and here's why: You burn a lot of carbs over 26.2 miles, so you want to pack as much as you can for the journey. Research confirms that it works. Several studies have shown that runners who eat more carbohydrates in the days prior to a marathon run faster times. So 3 days before the big day, increase your carbo-hydrate intake to around 4 grams per pound of body weight (some researchers advise going up to about 5.5 grams). To see what 4 grams per pound looks like, check out the chart opposite.

That's a lot of spaghetti. Where the heck does it all go? It gets stored as gly-cogen in your muscles and liver. The best strategy with carbo-loading before a race is the same as carbo-eating during your regular diet—spread it out over your day. You might also consider getting some of those carbs in the form of a high-protein sports beverage so you won't feel bloated and heavy.

In addition to carbo-loading, I do a little salt-loading before a marathon or triathlon. I learned first hand what happens when you lose too much salt in an event (you can read all about it on page 172), and I really don't want it to happen again. So the day before my race, I will put salt on my food and eat some salty pretzels. Yes, I know the American Heart Association is telling us we all

HUMPTY DUMPTY: LET'S HEAR IT FOR THE EGG

He may look like a buffoon, but underneath the thin shell of that teetering wall-sitter is a dietary superhero. Not only does the egg contain all nine essential amino acids (those that your body can-not make and which you must get from food), it has the highest biological value of protein of all foods, a measurement of the amount of protein that is actually used by the body. The egg is a good source of vitamins A and D, riboflavin, folate, and B_{12} (which is primarily found in meats). It also delivers lutein and zeaxanthin, which support good vision. Long vilified for its cholesterol con-tent (187 milligrams per egg; most of us should keep daily intake of cholesterol to 300 milligrams), the egg has earned the respect of experts every-where who now admire all that it has to offer and have altered their recommendations—an egg a day is A-okay.

CARBO-LOADING: 4 grams of carbs per pound of body weight per day

IF YOU WEIGH . . .	THAT'S THIS MANY GRAMS OF CARBS	THIS MANY CALORIES	AND THIS MANY CUPS OF COOKED SPAGHETTI
120 pounds	480	1,920	8½
130 pounds	520	2,080	9½
140 pounds	560	2,240	10
150 pounds	600	2,400	11
160 pounds	640	2,560	11½

need to cut way back on our salt intake, and I don't disagree. But I don't think the directive applies when you're running a marathon, especially on a hot, humid day. And whether it's salt-loading or carbo-loading, don't forget the golden rule: Try it out in training before you put it to the real test on race day.

Race Day

You would think after eating all those carbs you would be set for 26.2 miles, right? Unfortunately, that's not the case. If you manage to stuff carbs into every nook and cranny, that's 200 grams of glycogen in your liver plus 500 grams of glycogen in your muscles. It's enough to keep you going for about 2 hours or about 20 miles. In addition to eating whatever you would usually eat before a long run, you will need to refuel along the way. And believe me, I know; I have bonked in a lot of marathons. If you're not taking care of your nutrient needs during a long run or race, you could experience a whole spectrum of problems related to depletion. The first thing to go is sugar; you may feel weak, jittery, nauseated, or all of the above. Next up: dehydration, which causes muscle cramps and sluggishness. And

finally, if you lose too much salt, your muscles may cramp and you will feel disoriented.

What works for me in terms of carb replacement is to get about 200 to 250 calories (50 to 60 grams of carbohydrates) per hour, and research supports this. You can do this with either a sports beverage or a sports gel. It's a good idea to take in carbohydrate drinks or gels gradually over the course of the marathon so you don't upset your stomach. Aim to hit the water stops every 15 minutes and take 4 to 7 ounces of a sports beverage. If you prefer sports gels, take half an energy gel packet every 15 minutes with water or a whole packet every half hour, again with water to dilute it; a pile of concentrated sugar in your belly just might not sit well, if you know what I mean. I start taking carbs an hour to an hour and a half into an event, but sports nutritionists advise that you begin 30 minutes into your marathon. You know what I'm going to say next, don't you? Experiment in training during your long runs and figure out what works best for you. Though I have focused on marathons here, sports beverages or energy gels might give you an edge in a half-marathon as well.

A word about water: A loss of just 2 percent of your body weight as fluid—3 pounds if you weigh 150 pounds—diminishes your physical and mental performance by 20 percent. At 3 to 4 percent dehydration, your health is at risk. If you're sipping a sports drink every 15 minutes along the race course, you don't need to top if off with water. In fact, diluting the sports beverage will slow absorption of carbohydrates. If you choose not to take the sports drink at the stations along the race course, grab a cup of water instead.

Postrace Recovery

Congratulate yourself on completing your race. You should feel good about what you accomplished, even if you didn't run the time you had hoped.

You set a goal, trained hard, and ran the distance. Great job! As soon as you can after crossing the finish line, start replenishing spent carbohydrates, protein, and water using that same 4-to-1 ratio of carbs to protein that you use after a training run. Drink a sports beverage or maybe even some chocolate milk—anything that is good to replace depleted muscle glycogen stores and ensure a quicker turnaround before your next workout. Many call this period just after the workout a "golden half hour" where you can maximize nutritional replacement. While I don't think this is as essential as calling your mom or brushing your teeth, trying to get some replenishment within a half hour of the end of your workout is probably a good idea. And you will want to sit down to a full meal about 2 hours after you have crossed the finish line.

A FEW WORDS ABOUT WEIGHT LOSS

Some of you may run in order to manage your weight or because you want to drop a few pounds. And I have had new runners in particular tell me they have been running faithfully for weeks and feel really discouraged because

THE ELECTROLYTES—POTASSIUM AND SODIUM!

The electrolytes—sounds like the name of a '50s rock band, doesn't it? Well, potassium and sodium do rock for runners. And calcium is the third member of this trio that, when all are present and jamming in sync, brings on muscle contractions that rock 'n' roll you down the road. When sodium leaves the stage via sweat, however, muscles get grumpy and cramp up. Replace sodium and everyone's happy.

they haven't lost a pound. First, let me say that running is one of the most efficient ways to burn calories. Consider this: A 30-minute run at a 12-minute-per-mile pace burns twice as many calories as a 30-minute walk at a 17-minute pace. And if you throw some high-intensity intervals into that run (see Chapter 13 for details), you will burn even more. But let's say you are a 155-pound person looking to drop a few and you run 30 minutes a day at a 12-minute-per-mile pace. You will burn 293 calories with each 30 minute trek. Later that day you step into Starbucks and order a grande vanilla latte. At 250 calories a pop, it nearly wipes out your run—in terms of calories, that is. Here's another catch: Research shows that runners have a tendency to overestimate how many calories they have burned on a run, so they don't think twice about ordering that latte.

If you are one of the many who think they can take up running and then watch the pounds melt away, I'm sorry to say it doesn't quite work that way. You need to create a calorie deficit. You need to burn more calories than you consume, so you need to pay attention to your running mileage, running intensity, and what you eat.

One of my former patients, Grace (you can read her story on page 10), has a couple of diet tips that I think are so terrific I have to repeat them here: Eat a pile of green things whenever possible, and eat dessert only on Saturdays. As Grace points out in her story, you can eat a tremendous amount of green things without taking in a lot of calories (provided you haven't drenched those green things in high-fat dressings and sauces). And by eating dessert once a week, Grace cuts way back on empty calories without depriving herself. Her eating habits combined with her regular running trimmed 30 pounds from her frame in about 6 months.

Unlike Grace, I have not made any dietary decrees. I love to eat. I love food. And if I didn't exercise every day . . . well, I hate to think what my middle might look like. So I make good use of my metabolic furnace, and you can do the same. Exercise revs up metabolism and keeps it up even after you have stopped. It's the afterburn effect: When you stop exercising, you continue to stoke the furnace and burn calories at a higher rate than you would normally at rest, and the greater the intensity of your workout, the hotter the afterburn. I run first thing in the morning before work to turn my metabolic furnace on high for the day. When I'm having dinner in the city after work, I will take my running clothes to the office, and at the end of the day, I change, slip on my backpack, and head out of the office for my running commute home.

You will find plenty of great weight-loss tools for runners on runnersworld.com, including a calculator that tells you how many calories you burned on your run. By playing around with how far you run, how fast you run, when you run, and what you eat, you can trim down to the weight that's right for you and your best health.

MY RECIPE FOR HEALTHY EATING

There's tons of great information available about foods and the nutrients they provide and about how to build a nutritious diet. A terrific source is the Web site of the Academy of Nutrition and Dietetics, eatright.org, and we are sure to hear more from sports nutrition scientists as they continue to explore ways that diet can help us run faster and farther. But for now, here's what works for me, and what I believe can help you run your healthiest and your best.

1. Eat what you love and love what you eat.

2. Pile lots of veggies and whole grains on your plate, followed by lean proteins and healthy fats.

3. Drink water until your pee is nearly clear.

4. Keep in mind that a few fries will not kill you.

5. Go ahead and have dessert. Just don't make it your main source of carbs.

6. Fuel up before and during long runs and races.

7. Replenish spent carbohydrates, protein, and water for an excellent recovery.

Bon appétit!

EAT BEETS TO BEAT YOUR RIVALS

Yep, beets—baked beets.

Scientists know that nitrate improves athletic performance, but it also has negative health effects unless consumed in vegetables. To explore whether a high-nitrate veggie, like beets, could boost running times, researchers at Saint Louis University recruited 11 moderately fit men and women to run two separate 5-K time trials on a treadmill. Seventy-five minutes prior to one of two 5-Ks, the runners ate 200 grams of baked beets (equal to two beets about 2 inches in diameter), which contains 500 milligrams of nitrate. Seventy-five minutes prior to the other 5-K, those same men and women ate the same number of calories in cranberry relish (the placebo). And you guessed it: Beets won. After eating baked beets, the runners ran 5 percent faster for the last mile of the 5-K than after eating the placebo, shaving a whopping 41 seconds off their race times.

You might want to consider making beets the secret weapon before your next race. Hate beets? Leafy greens—including Swiss chard, beet greens, spring greens, and arugula—have even more nitrate. Arugula, in fact, has twice the nitrate content, delivering 960 milligrams in 200 grams (7 ounces). Eat those greens!

CHAPTER 16

GOOD SHOES and COOL CLOTHES

Choosing a pair of running shoes is the most important decision you will make as a runner.

A patient of mine once said, "My choice of running shoe is more important than my choice of spouse." Well, I wouldn't say it's quite *that* important, but getting in the right pair of shoes really makes a huge difference to your running experience. It will affect every step you take. A quarter of your body's bones are in your feet—26 per foot, 52 in a pair. Treat those babies with care. Get them a pair of running shoes that they will love. I'll show you how.

HEAD OVER HEELS: THE BAREFOOT DEBATE

But, Dr. Metzl, do I even need running shoes, you ask? That question has been debated ever since the debut of Christopher McDougall's book *Born to Run* in 2009, which turned our eyes to our soles and made us question whether we would be healthier and faster runners without them. There's a great case to be made for running barefoot.

1. It strengthens your feet and ankles because both have to work harder without the crutch of a pair of shoes to support them. Stronger feet and ankles are less prone to injury.

2. Running shoes encourage a rear-foot landing, which may make you more prone to injury. And why is that? Your foot is farther out in front during a rear-foot landing and your leg is straighter, so you "brake" as you land, and that braking action increases the stress up your leg.

3. Barefoot running shifts the landing to your midfoot. Your foot hits the ground beneath your body, beneath your center of mass. There is no braking action. In addition, you bend more at the knee; your leg mechanically has more flexibility, and your body does a better job of absorbing the force of impact.

4. When you land on your midfoot, you spend less time on the ground in the stance phase of running. Running economy improves, which may mean faster race times.

Sounds like barefoot running is the way to go, right?

Here's the But

Before you toss your trainers in the trash, let me ask you this: Have you worn shoes most of your life and running shoes most of your running life? If you answered yes, hold on to those trainers. Think back to our discussion in Chapter 13: Your brain is an eager learner. It wants to help you live your healthiest life. So though you were born barefoot, once you started wearing shoes, your brain began working with your muscles to learn how to walk and then run in shoes, and by now, many years later, your entire kinetic chain has become expert at it. If you decide you're going to start running au naturel today, not only might you cut your foot on a stone or scrap of glass lying in the road, but you also risk muscular injury, particularly of the Achilles tendon and calf muscles, which have to work in ways they are not accustomed to, ways that they haven't learned.

Even shifting all your training to a minimalist shoe is a little risky. The value of barefoot running is to get you into a shorter, faster stride—170 to 180 footstrikes per minute is ideal. So here's what I recommend if you want to try minimalist shoes: Use them for shorter runs and then translate that running style and form to your regular shoes. In other words, train your mind and body how to shorten your stride and keep your weight balanced over your feet by using minimalist shoes, and then use this style with your normal shoes. Only very few people can run big miles in minimalist shoes without getting injured, but we can all benefit from the stylistic advantages that this type of shoe offers.

By the way, in addition to cadence, another important reason to keep your tried-and-true trainers on is that the right shoe can help correct foot-motion problems that could lead to injury. So you see, this is never a one-size-fits-all decision.

STEP INTO MY OFFICE

Blipp this page to view a video about how to select the running shoe that's right for you.

HOW TO CHOOSE THE RIGHT SHOE FOR YOU

Running shoes are designed to protect your feet from sticks and stones and prevent injury by steering your foot motion toward the ideal. If Goldilocks were a runner, she would have just the right amount of foot motion—not too much, not too little, just right.

We talked about foot motion way back in Chapter 2, but let's have a quick review.

- Your foot strikes the ground on the outside toward your heel.
- Your arch lowers as your foot rolls inward toward the center.
- You move forward on your foot toward your big toe and push off.

What I have just described is just right. It's normal pronation for a runner with a neutral foot, and this motions helps you best absorb the force of impact. If you overpronate, your foot rolls inward too far when you land, and that puts extra strain on the inside of your ankle and shin and can cause shin splints and iliotibial band syndrome (if you haven't watched my video, please do; this will all make a lot more sense when I show you on a live human being). If you underpronate, your foot doesn't roll inward enough; it remains stiff and rigid and can't cushion the blow of impact. This lack of motion makes you more vulnerable to stress injuries and fractures.

So your first step in finding your perfect shoe is to look at your foot motion, which, clearly, you can't do on your own. Have someone—a physical therapist or a knowledgeable salesperson at your local running shop—watch you walk barefoot.

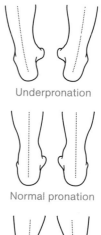

Underpronation

Normal pronation

Overpronation

If, like Goldilocks, your foot motion is just right, simply choose the shoes that feel most comfortable on your feet and that fit properly. If you overpronate, check out motion-control shoes. These have a medial post—an area of denser material built into the midsole along the inner, or medial, side of the shoe that helps prevent your foot from rolling too far inward as you run. If you underpronate, steer clear of motion-control shoes. You want *more* movement. You also want more cushioning since your stiff, rigid foot is slamming hard into the ground with every stride. Look for shoes that have plenty of cushioning and no medial post in the midsole.

These are simply guidelines to finding a great shoe. The most important attributes you need in your running shoes are comfort and fit. If the salesperson brings you a few models to try and you're not loving any of them, don't be afraid to try on more.

I'm an overpronator and I used to get shin splints and iliotibial band syndrome, so I wore a heavier motion-control shoe for years. But I have an increasing belief that it's not just what's going on between your shoe and the road that matters. It's equally important to know what's going on inside the shoe—between the shoe and your foot. Here's what I mean by that: I have changed my shoe from a heavier motion-control shoe to a lighter, more neutral shoe with a heat-

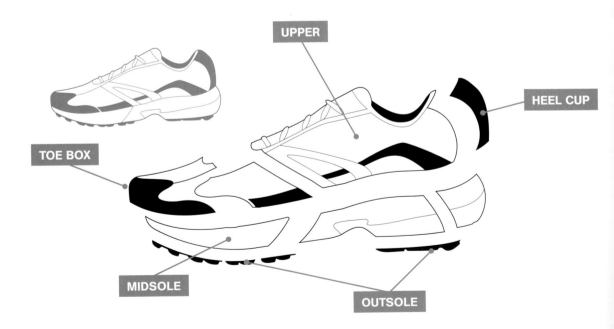

UPPER

HEEL CUP

TOE BOX

MIDSOLE

OUTSOLE

moldable orthotic. The lighter shoe is more comfortable and makes me a more efficient runner. And the orthotic supports my foot motion so that I don't get injured.

I have runners come into my office all the time with injuries caused by lousy foot motion, and they will say, "But my running store told me this is the shoe I needed." First, let me say that I love specialty running stores and I think most of the personnel are very well informed. But I don't believe in a one-size-fits-all solution. If your motion-control shoe is working fine, great. But maybe you are someone who overpronates and who, like me, would prefer a neutral shoe and an over-the-counter orthotic. Don't feel pressured to take the one solution that's offered up to you. This is an individual choice. You need to decide what feels comfortable, what feels right for you.

Shoe Shopping

Ready to go buy your perfect pair of running shoes? Well, it might take a little trial and error to find your number one, but keeping in mind that the two most important qualities in a running shoe are comfort and fit, here's how to make sure your shoes have both.

1. Shop at a specialty running store. It will have the best selection and the best expertise in making sure the fit is right.

2. Shop in the late afternoon or early evening. Your feet swell a little bit throughout the day just as they will during a run, so you want to try on shoes with your feet at their largest.

3. Don't be afraid to try a lot of different shoes to find what's most comfortable.

4. Check for these fit factors.
   a. Snug around the heel
   b. A thumb's width of space between your longest toe (which might be your second toe) and the top of the shoe
   c. Snug but not tight in the toe box (your toes should have a little room to wiggle)

WET SHOES

Remember as a kid how you loved to run through puddles? For the kid inside you, it may still be a lot of fun, but soggy midsoles have 40 to 50 percent less shock-absorbing capability than dry ones, so skirt around those puddles. If you can't avoid them or if you get caught in a downpour on your run, let your shoes air-dry. Don't toss them in the dryer; the heat can break down the midsole and its components and shorten the life of your shoes.

5. Take them for a test run. Running stores will let you use their treadmill if they have one or go out to the street for a short run. Focus on the fit.

   a. Your heel should not slip up and down; if it does, you will get blisters.

   b. Your toe should not bang against the front of the shoe—unless you happen to like the look of black toenails.

   c. The shoes should feel snug; your feet shouldn't be sliding around inside like the cargo on a ship traveling through rough seas.

   d. Specifics aside, do the shoes feel comfortable on your feet? Ask yourself, is this the right running shoe for me?

6. Choose function over fashion. I know, there are a lot of really cool-looking running shoes on the market these days, but go for what works; don't worry about what it looks like.

Many running shops will let you return shoes if you have worn them for a few runs and find they're just not as comfortable as you thought. Ask the store about its return policy.

Again, if you're shopping for your first pair of running shoes or if the model you have loved for years has been discontinued, it might take a little trial and error to find your perfect fit. Don't be afraid to experiment. Maybe you need to add an orthotic to the shoe you currently wear, or maybe, like me, you will be happiest in a lighter neutral shoe plus an insert. If your feet love the shoes you have been wearing and you have been injury free, hey, congratulations, keep on running in them.

COOL CLOTHES

Today's running clothes look cool, but more importantly, they keep you cool, which during a hot and humid race can literally be a lifesaver. I know runners who swear by cotton. They love the way it feels and that it's a natural fiber. Cotton does a great job of absorbing sweat from your skin, but it holds on to that moisture, making you feel like a wet rag. My advice? Keep the cotton tees in your dresser drawer for casual nonathletic occasions and pull out running gear made from moisture-wicking fabrics, such as Coolmax, Dri-FIT, and drirelease. These polyester fabrics are designed with microfibers that wick moisture away from your skin to the surface of the fabric where it evaporates. You know the equation: Evaporation equals cooling. So choose tops, shorts, socks, bras, running tights, and jackets made from breathable, moisture-wicking fabrics. They are more expensive, yes, but worth the cost in comfort, coolness, and even quicker race times.

The Well-Dressed Runner

When the temperature and humidity soar, we all know what to wear—as little as possible. Once the weather turns cooler, many runners—especially those who are just starting out, but even seasoned runners—will scan the weather on their smartphones and then do the dance of decision. Is it too cool for a tank top? Short sleeves or long? Do I need a jacket? Once you have done this dance several times before a training run and run in any number of combinations of tops and bottoms, you will probably figure out how to dress for comfort in all types of weather.

The biggest mistake runners make is overdressing for the cold. It's easy to underestimate just how much you will warm up after a mile or more. Some runners have it figured out, and they step out on a 40-degree day in a T-shirt and shorts, endure a chilly mile or two, and then warm up to their perfect temperature. Others would rather not suffer even one mile of goose bumps, and I'm one of those runners. The solution? Layering. I am an expert at layering. Depending on how cold it is, I will wear two or three layers—a long-sleeve tee over short sleeves and, on really cold days, a jacket on top. As

I warm up, I peel off the outer layer and simply tie it around my waist. How you dress for running is as individual as the shoes you lace up on your feet. Experiment and you will become expert in what's most comfortable for you in any weather.

Limiting Bounce: The Sports Bra

Even if you don't have a lot to bounce during a run, too much movement stretches the Cooper's ligaments that support your breasts, which can eventually lead to sagging. That aside, bouncing is just plain uncomfortable, and for women with large breasts, it can be so painful that they will choose not to exercise at all. So keep breast movement to a minimum with a good sports bra, or maybe even two.

There are two broad categories of bras: the compression type, which essentially holds your breasts close to your chest, and the encapsulated style, which separates and supports each breast individually. Encapsulated bras offer the best support, and though any woman can wear them, if you are a size C cup or larger, you seriously want to consider this style. Compression bras should really only be worn by As and Bs. As with any piece of athletic apparel, the best bra is the one that fits well and feels comfortable.

Apparently finding a comfortable, well-fitting bra isn't that easy. In a survey of women who ran the 2012 London

Marathon, 75 percent reported that their bras had caused problems during the race. The top two complaints were chafing and straps digging into their shoulders. So how do you find a comfortable, supportive bra that fits well? This is one area of running where I don't have firsthand knowledge, but here's what my patients tell me.

1. Shop at a running store, where you will find a variety of models designed specifically for running.

2. Try on multiple brands.

3. Take multiple sizes into the dressing room for each model that you try on. If you think you're a medium, grab a small and a large. Different styles and models fit differently. Also, your body changes as you get older, after having children, and then again when you go through menopause.

4. The straps should lay flat and feel snug but not tight; they shouldn't slide along your shoulder or dig in.

5. The band should fit snugger than the band on your day-to-day bra—a band that is too loose will cause chafing—but it should still feel comfortable around your chest.

6. The bra should fit smoothly across your chest; if you see puckering or creasing in the fabric, you may need to go down a size.

7. Your breasts should be completely contained within the bra. If they're popping out the sides or top, you probably need to go up a size.

THE WET TEST

Runners have been doing this self-test for years: Wet your feet and stand on a flat, dry surface that will show your wet footprint. If your footprint is completely filled in, you have flat feet; if you see a really deep curve in your footprint, you have high arches. An average curve means you have an average or neutral foot. Generally speaking, a flat foot is associated with overpronation, a deep curve with under-pronation, and a middle-of-the-road curve suggests a normal foot. But though the wet test is a good indicator of the height of your arch, it does not define your foot motion during running. For that you need a knowledgeable person—a physical therapist, coach, or staff person at your running store—to watch you walk barefoot.

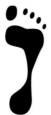 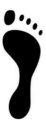 

DO YOU NEED ORTHOTICS?

Let's say you're plagued by iliotibial band syndrome and shin splints. You learn that you are an overpronator, so you buy a highly rated motion-control shoe. But you still get injured. The next step is to try an insert or orthotic. I find that most people don't need custom orthotics, which are very expensive. You can pick up over-the-counter orthotics at your local running shop, and they will do the job for most runners. I like heat-moldable orthotics, which you can find online. They are the same price as the inserts sold at your local running store, and several companies make them. You buy them, heat them up, and then they mold to your feet. How cool is that?

8. If everything looks good, jog in place and jump up and down to evaluate the bra's support and comfort.

9. And you have heard this advice from me before: Don't try anything new on race day. You don't want to be one of those London marathoners who endured the discomfort of a poor-fitting sports bra for miles and miles. Wear your new bra on your long runs to make sure it's not going to give you any problems on race day.

The Lowly but Highly Important Sock

I have two words for you when it comes to choosing socks: fit and breathability. Remember, you have about 250,000 sweat glands in each foot. Let that moisture out. Skip the cotton and go for the breathable synthetics. And pick the right size for your foot. Your socks shouldn't feel tight, but they should be snug, because if they bunch up inside your shoe, you're looking at a high probability of blisters, especially if you're running long. And speaking of blisters, my preference is to apply some moisturizer on blister-prone spots before I put on my socks, but some runners swear by double-layer socks.

And other runners swear by compression socks, but not for blister prevention. The thinking is that these socks increase bloodflow, which speeds recovery after a hard workout or race and, during speedwork or racing, sweeps lactic acid out of your muscles faster, allowing metabolism to continue at a good pace. There have been a few studies that show some positive effect of compression socks on recovery, but more research needs to be done to build a solid case. There is no evidence that they are harmful, so if you want to give them a try, go ahead. Just make sure you do what's comfortable and try to be an honest judge as to how well these socks work for you.

A SHOUT-OUT TO SUN PROTECTION

Plenty of evidence exists showing a higher incidence of melanoma—the deadliest form of skin cancer—among runners than among nonrunners, which is why I would like to give a shout-out to skin care. Please don't run without sunscreen. I like the ones that contain zinc oxide. They provide better protection from UVA rays, and they don't break down in sunlight. Use a cream rather than a spray; you will get better coverage. Apply a full ounce over every millimeter of exposed skin, and reapply every 2 hours. The studies that report a high incidence of skin cancer among runners also note that about half of the runners who were part of the study didn't use any sunscreen. Don't let that be you. And if you're a guy who's losing his hair, wear a hat when you run.

It's also important to protect your eyes when you're running in strong sunlight, and even during winter runs on bright, snowy days when there's lots of glare coming off the snow. Choose lenses that provide 100 percent protection from both UVA and UVB light. Wraparound glasses will block light that's coming from the sides. I like lighter sports sunglasses with a longer earpiece that fits snug so my specs stay put. I'm also a big fan of visors, which help shade my face from bright sun. Choose what feels right to you. Just be sure to choose to use sun protection when you run.

PART V

His and Hers

At the finish line, the race goes to the fastest—man or woman. But along the way, we each have our own stuff to deal with. Let's figure it out together.

CHAPTER 17
GENDER DIFFERENCES

Running is an equal-opportunity activity. That's why I love recommending it to kids, teens, and adults as part of my exercise prescription. Anyone—young or old, thin or overweight, fit or unfit, man or woman—can run and improve and stay healthy and injury-free for years and years. And people of all abilities are welcome in any road race anywhere in the world. What sport is more welcoming? You gotta love it!

But of course, not all runners are equal. And though a man and a woman can line up right next to each other at the start of a 5-K and even cross the finish line at the same time, they face different challenges or potential challenges as determined by their chromosomes. So let's look at those differences and what it means for your running and your health.

HER WORLD

To all the women reading this book, let me start by saying I'm not you, but at least from a medical perspective, I get you—your running and nonrunning lives are, generally speaking, a bit more complex than men's. You endure a flux of hormones not just monthly but throughout your life—puberty, pregnancy, and menopause. Your body is constantly changing (we will look at what that means for you as a runner). And then there's life: Most of you still juggle more of the home, work, and family responsibilities, and your nurturing nature seems to guide you to put all of these in front of your own needs.

Finally, let's be honest: Society puts a lot of pressure on you to be thin—too thin. The pressure on women to be skinny, and not a healthy slim, is a problem. I'm thrilled to see that there's a lot of backlash against the unattainable female body images we see in the media, but those images are still everywhere, and they still drive women to feel bad about themselves. Combine the societal pressure to be thin with a sport that favors a lean body, and a female runner might just go too far in her quest for the "perfect" body and find herself caught in the female-athlete triad, a cascade of events that can lead to the cessation of menstruation and bone loss. We will talk about that in detail, but let's start with something much less consequential.

The Q-Angle

We all have one—women and men. The Q-angle, or quadriceps angle, is the angle of your quadriceps relative to your kneecap. If you were to take a piece of string and stretch it straight up your leg from the center of your kneecap to the top of your thigh, and then you took a second piece of string and, starting at that same point in the center of your kneecap, stretched it to the outside of your hip, the angle in between is your Q-angle (see the illustration opposite). Why does this come up more often when we're talking about female runners? Because, generally speaking, women have wider pelvises and therefore bigger Q-angles.

So? Well, if you remember back to Chapter 2, your quadriceps play a key role in stabilizing your knee and making sure it operates like a well-oiled hinge, moving straight up and down. When your quads are working at a greater angle away from your knee, they put more strain on your kneecap, which over time can lead to patellofemoral knee pain, or runner's knee. And I can tell you I see this injury more often among my female patients than my male ones.

What to do about it? The answer is simple: strength and flexibility. The quadriceps, remember, are a group of muscles, and in some runners the inner muscle, the vastus medialis, may be weak. Squats are a great strengthener. Also, you want to keep the muscles in your legs flexible because tight muscles create more tension. If you're doing the IronStrength workout regularly and using your foam roller every day,

you're good; your Q-angle shouldn't cause you any trouble. If you're not using those programs, please turn to Chapter 12.

The Female-Athlete Triad

This is the Bermuda triangle of women's running. I've known runners to get caught in it and have a really difficult time getting out. The triad is a serious threat to a woman's health. The danger begins with calorie restriction. Some female runners slide into it unintentionally. They set a goal to train for a marathon, for example, and as they put in more miles and add some more intensity to their training, they simply

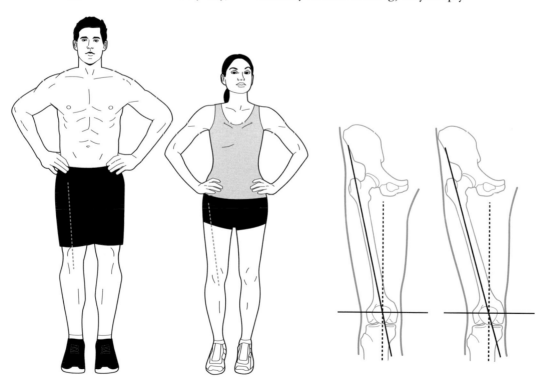

On average, women have a greater Q-angle than men do.

neglect to add more food to their diet, so they lose weight. One day they notice that they're a lot thinner. And they think thin is good, right? You have less weight to carry with you when you run, and you're on your way to achieving a fashion model's figure. So they say to themselves, "Look at me—I lost weight without even trying. I'm going to make sure I don't gain an ounce back. In fact, if I watch what I eat, maybe I can lose even more." It doesn't help that in the beginning you get positive feedback from faster race times as well as friends and family who notice that you have lost weight. You're cruising straight for the triad: calorie deficiency + menstrual malfunction + bone loss.

When you don't take in enough calories to nourish your body, one of the first bodily systems to shut down is menstruation. The menstrual cycle gets longer and irregular, and if calorie deprivation continues or increases, menstruation will eventually just stop.

Three or more consecutive months of missed periods is called amenorrhea, and if that defines your current menstrual status, see your doctor. Girls who consume too few calories may delay the onset of menstruation, and if a girl hasn't had her first period by the time she is 16, she needs to see a doctor.

When menstruation grinds to a halt, estrogen levels take a dive—and that's bad news for your bones. Bone tissue is constantly being remodeled: It's tapped to provide calcium for the rest of your body, and then it's built back up. Estrogen prevents bone from being broken down faster than it can be rebuilt. Take estrogen out of the equation and you have bone loss. It's easy to see why women who are amenorrheic are at a much higher risk of stress fractures and even osteoporosis.

Loss of calories means loss of nutrition. Your health begins to fail, and so does your running. In the early stages of the triad, you may not notice any negative effect on performance, but as

RUNNING CIRCLES AROUND YOUR CYCLE

Like it or not, female runners train on hills every month. I'm not talking about the ones you climb on your road runs—rather, your hormonal ups and downs. Some days, for no good reason it seems, you feel sluggish and fatigued and running is hard. Other days you have a spring in your step. And though there might be any number of reasons for your energy or lack thereof, one possibility is your menstrual cycle. Because every woman responds differently to her personal ebb and flow of hor-

mones, keep a log of how you feel when you run and also note where you are in your cycle. Once you have found a pattern, take advantage of it. Schedule some intense training for those days when you know you will feel frisky, and keep it short and sweet when the going gets rough.

Do cramps and bloating dampen your desire to run? Just go anyway. Most women tell me they are surprised to find that running makes them feel better and gives them a boost of energy.

calorie deprivation continues, training gets tougher, you fatigue more easily, and your race times fall. The solution is simple: Eat enough calories and the right foods to feed your health and fuel your running. Unfortunately, it's not so simple for the woman who struggles with body image or an unrealistic pursuit of better performances through thinness or who gets seduced by the false sense of control she may feel when she limits what she eats. But there is always a way out, and a team of professionals—a coach, a nutritionist, and a therapist—can help her find her way back to good health.

The tricky thing here is that the female-athlete triad can happen at any age but is most common in adolescent and college-age athletes. The problem is that by the age of 32, you have made all the bone you are going to make ever; you have reached your peak bone mass. So if a young woman gets caught in the female-athlete triad, she may not achieve the bone growth that she would have if she were healthy, which greatly increases her risk for osteoporosis later in life.

When it comes to the female-athlete triad, the best defense is a good offense. Prevent it from happening in the first place. Pay attention to signs: A BMI under 21, missed periods, and stress fractures all indicate that you are heading down an unhealthy path. Stop. See your doctor and discuss what's going on before it becomes difficult to turn back.

Running During and After Pregnancy

Some of you reading this may be several years away from having a baby; others may be pregnant and running (or not); and there are those of you who just had a baby and are looking to get back to running or are running already. First, let me say this: If you want to run or are running during your pregnancy, I support you 100 percent. It's safe for you and your baby, and it can make your pregnancy easier and more enjoyable. Running helps you maintain a healthy weight, prevent gestational diabetes, maintain your cardiovascular fitness and endurance, boost your energy, improve sleep, and reduce backache, and it will put you in a good mood. So you have lots of great reasons to run during pregnancy. But if you aren't a runner, this isn't the best time to start. Even if you are, make sure you talk about your plans to run with your obstetrician. If your pregnancy falls in the high-risk category, your doctor may suggest some alternatives to running. Regardless, your doc needs to know your exercise plans.

Now, let's talk about what you can expect when you're expecting. You will probably notice, even in the early weeks, that running feels a little harder than usual, almost like you're running for two. You will run slower and fatigue earlier because your cardiovascular and respiratory systems have to work harder to deliver blood and oxygen to both your body and your developing fetus. Then come the bio-mechanical changes. In the second trimester, as your baby bump grows, your center of gravity shifts; by week 13 your body starts producing the hormone relaxin, which relaxes ligaments and joints throughout your body for the eventual delivery of your baby. Both of these phenomena up your odds of injury, so you need to be more mindful of how you feel when you run and what kind of running you do. This is not the best time to do any challenging trail runs.

What are the rules of the road if you decide to run during your pregnancy? I don't have any personal experience to add to this one, but here's my professional advice.

1. **Be consistent.** Plan to run at least 30 minutes 3 days a week. This doesn't mean you can't go longer. Did you regularly hit 40 miles each week before you got pregnant? Go for it.

2. **Put your pace in its place.** Go slow to moderate, 60 to 85 percent of your max heart rate.

3. **Eat for one-plus.** You're not eating for two, so please don't double your food intake. But do double your efforts to eat healthy foods: lean proteins, low-fat dairy, lots of fruits and veggies, and whole grains. And drink plenty of water. During pregnancy your body needs more calcium, iron, and folate. Your doc will prescribe a prenatal vitamin, but you should continue to get most of your calories from nutrient-rich, low-fat foods. Does this mean you shouldn't satisfy a craving? By all means, if your partner is willing to drive to the nearest convenience store in the middle of the night for Ben & Jerry's Cherry Garcia, go ahead and have some; just don't eat the whole pint.

4. **Stick to even surfaces.** After your first trimester, your ligaments begin to loosen and your center of gravity

STOP SIGNS FOR THE PREGNANT RUNNER

The American Congress of Obstetricians and Gynecologists advises that you stop running and call your doctor. if you experience any of the following symptoms.

- Vaginal bleeding
- Dizziness or feeling faint
- Increased shortness of breath
- Chest pain
- Headache
- Muscle weakness
- Calf pain or swelling
- Uterine contractions
- Decreased fetal movement
- Fluid leaking from the vagina

starts to shift. Run where the terrain won't twist your ankle or trip you up.

5. **Keep your cool.** Plan your hot-day runs for early morning or evening, when the temperatures are cooler. Wear light clothing and drink plenty of water. If it's too hot and humid for you to run comfortably outdoors, consider running on a treadmill or in a pool, or taking the day off.

6. **Plan for pit stops.** As your uterus grows, so does the pressure on your bladder. Try to map a run that takes you past a public restroom or two.

7. **Seek support.** If your growing belly makes running uncomfortable, consider wearing a support belt. You can find them online.

8. **Follow what feels right.** As your pregnancy progresses, you will probably naturally cut back on mileage and pace. This is not the time to be chasing personal bests. You are running for health. If what you're doing doesn't feel healthy, cut back or switch to swimming or walking.

9. **Adjust your IronStrength workouts as needed.** You can continue with IronStrength, but after the first trimester, no more exercises on your back (crunches, legs up) and no jumping. You will also probably want to cut back on the number of sets for each exercise as your

pregnancy moves forward. Do what feels comfortable—physically, physiologically, and psychologically.

If there is ever a time to listen to your body as a female runner, this is it. There is no prescription for how many miles or what pace you should run. Elite distance runners will be able to tolerate higher mileage and intensities than moderately competitive runners or women who run for fun and fitness. Some women choose to run only through the first trimester; others run up until the third; still others run until they give birth. Then there are those women who choose not to run at all during pregnancy—and that's cool too. Listen to your body and mind. You need to make the decision that feels right for you. Let physical and mental comfort guide you.

And that goes for your return to running after pregnancy. Some women can hit the road running right after they have delivered a baby, and that's fine if that's you, but that very well might not be you. Begin when you feel ready. If you chose not to run during your pregnancy or you stopped after the first or second trimester, walk first, then progress to a walk/run, and finally continuous runs as you feel ready. If you had a C-section or a difficult vaginal birth, it's a good idea to talk with your doctor about when to start exercising again.

HIS WORLD

Stinky feet and bloody nipples—gross, right? Welcome to the world of the male runner. With about 3,000 sweat glands to every square inch of foot, we men produce the lion's share of foot odor. Given the poor performance of the olfactory sense, we might not even notice, but anyone who comes near us—if they even get near us—will. Guys, we would probably be wise to follow in the steps of women when it comes to our feet and show our stinky dogs a little love: regular bathing, thorough drying, a dusting of baby powder, and a fresh pair of moisture-wicking socks daily. Do not—I repeat, do not—pick up yesterday's running socks off the floor to wear during today's 10-miler. For more tips on how to tame the stink, turn to Chapter 11.

In that same chapter, you will find strategies to prevent another common male runner's malady—bloody nipples, due to constant chafing against your tee during long, hot, sweaty runs. Give me stinky feet any day over the sting of raw nipples at mile 20 of a marathon. But this, too, is preventable: Nip-Guards—just get 'em.

Hey, I love humor and am happy to joke around with you about your feet, but the biggest concern I have for male runners is not a laughing matter—it's your risk of cardiac arrest during half-marathons and marathons. Now, before your heart skips a beat over that statement, let me reassure you that your risk of having a heart attack during a long-distance race is *extremely* low. For proof, we have the biggest study ever to examine risk of cardiac events during long-distance races.

A group of physicians called the Race Associated Cardiac Arrest Event Registry Study Group, headed by Dr. Jonathan H. Kim of Harvard Medical School, examined the incidence of cardiac arrest in men and women who had completed half- and full marathons from January 1, 2000, to May 31, 2010.[1] That's a lot of runners— 10.9 million to be exact. And of those 10.9 million runners, a mere 59 had cardiac arrest. Here are some of the key findings.

- 40 of the heart attacks occurred during a marathon

- 19 occurred during a half-marathon

- 51 of the 59 runners (86 percent) who suffered cardiac arrest were men

- 42 of the 59 runners (71 percent) died

- The mean age of those who died: 39

---

1. Kim, J. H., R. Malhotra, G. Chiampas, P. d'Hemecourt, C. Troyanos , J. Cianca , R. N. Smith, et al., "Cardiac Arrest during Long-Distance Running Races," *New England Journal of Medicine* 366, no. 2 (January 2012): 130–40.

- The mean age of those who survived: 49

- The most common cause of death: hypertrophic cardiomyopathy

What the heck is hypertrophic cardiomyopathy (HCM), you ask? It's when one part of your heart muscle, usually the left ventricle, is thicker than the other parts, and this thickening means your heart must work harder to move blood out of the heart and to relax and fill with blood. Bottom line is that bloodflow is reduced. In most cases, HCM is inherited. It is the most common cause of sudden cardiac death in young athletes in any sport, and it can go undetected for years. If you know that someone in your family had or has HCM or if you experience any of the following symptoms, see a cardiologist for a complete evaluation.

- Chest pain that occurs with running or at rest

- Unusual shortness of breath when running

- Dizziness or fainting with running

- Heart palpitations or fluttering

The treatment for HCM depends on many factors and might include medication or a defibrillator, or even a surgical procedure. Most runners diagnosed with this heart condition will be able to continue to run, although probably not competitively.

Scary stuff, I know. But remember, we're talking about 59 heart attacks among 10.9 million runners. The risk is very low. And the flip side of all of this is that running *protects* you from heart disease—big time. Science shows over and over again that long-distance runners, including marathoners, have lower weight, lower blood pressure and heart rate, lower levels of triglycerides (fats) in the bloodstream, higher levels of HDL cholesterol (the good kind), and overall a significantly lower risk of heart disease when compared with sedentary or even minimally active men and women. So don't hesitate to lace up your running shoes and go the long distance.

I'll see you on the road.

APPENDIX

OFF to the RACES

Sometimes we run races just for the fun of it, and we really don't care about how fast we finish. But let's be honest, most of the time when we're packed behind the starting line of an event, we are chomping at the bit to do our best.

To help you do just that, I asked *Runner's World* magazine coach Budd Coates to design training templates for every kind of runner, from the first-timer to the seasoned speedy competitor. Here are week-by-week schedules for the 5-K, 10-K, half-marathon, and marathon that show how many miles to run, when to run them, and how to plug in IronStrength and cross-training. All of these schedules include two quality workouts a week—a long run on Sunday and speedwork or hills on Wednesday (for more information about different types of speed training, see Chapter 13).

Now, ready, set, go!

THE 5-K

Beginner: Just Getting Started

WEEK	MONDAY	TUESDAY	WEDNESDAY	THURSDAY	FRIDAY	SATURDAY	SUNDAY
1	0 or cross-train	3	4	IronStrength	3	0 or cross-train	4
2	0 or cross-train	3	4	IronStrength	3	0 or cross-train	4
3	0 or cross-train	3	5	IronStrength	3	0 or cross-train	5
4	0 or cross-train	4	5	IronStrength	4	0 or cross-train	5–6
5	0 or cross-train	4	5	IronStrength	4	0 or cross-train	6
6	0 or cross-train	4	6	IronStrength	4	0 or cross-train	6
7	0 or cross-train	3	6	IronStrength	4	0 or cross-train	4
8	0 or cross-train	3	4	0–2	0	2	5-K

Intermediate: Moving Up

WEEK	MONDAY	TUESDAY	WEDNESDAY	THURSDAY	FRIDAY	SATURDAY	SUNDAY
1	0–2 or cross-train	4	6	IronStrength	3	0 or cross-train	6–8
2	0–2 or cross-train	4	6	IronStrength	3	0 or cross-train	6
3	0–2 or cross-train	4	6	IronStrength	0–4	0 or cross-train	8
4	0–2 or cross-train	4–6	6	IronStrength	0–4	0 or cross-train	6
5	0–2 or cross-train	4–6	7–8	IronStrength	0–4	0 or cross-train	8–10
6	0–2 or cross-train	4	7–8	IronStrength	0–4	0 or cross-train	6
7	0–2 or cross-train	4	6	IronStrength	4	0 or cross-train	6
8	0–2 or cross-train	4	6	0–2	0	2	5-K

Advanced: At the Front of the Pack

WEEK	MONDAY	TUESDAY	WEDNESDAY	THURSDAY	FRIDAY	SATURDAY	SUNDAY
1	0–2 or cross-train	4–6	6	IronStrength	4	0–3 or cross-train	6–8
2	0–2 or cross-train	4–6	6	IronStrength	4	0–3 or cross-train	6
3	0–2 or cross-train	4–6	6	IronStrength	5	0–3 or cross-train	8–10
4	0–2 or cross-train	6	7–8	IronStrength	5	0–3 or cross-train	6
5	0–2 or cross-train	6	7–8	IronStrength	5	0–3 or cross-train	8–10
6	0–2 or cross-train	6	7–8	IronStrength	4	0 or cross-train	6
7	0–2 or cross-train	4–6	7–8	IronStrength	4	0–2 or cross-train	6–8
8	0–2 or cross-train	4	6	0–2	0	2	5-K

THE 10-K

Beginner: Just Getting Started

WEEK	MONDAY	TUESDAY	WEDNESDAY	THURSDAY	FRIDAY	SATURDAY	SUNDAY
1	0 or cross-train	3	4	IronStrength	3	0 or cross-train	6
2	0 or cross-train	3	4	IronStrength	3	0 or cross-train	6
3	0 or cross-train	3	4	IronStrength	3	0 or cross-train	7–8
4	0 or cross-train	4	5	IronStrength	3	0 or cross-train	6
5	0 or cross-train	4–5	5	IronStrength	4	0 or cross-train	8
6	0 or cross-train	4–5	5	IronStrength	4–5	0 or cross-train	6
7	0 or cross-train	4–5	6	IronStrength	4–5	0 or cross-train	8
8	0 or cross-train	4	6	IronStrength	4	0 or cross-train	6
9	0 or cross-train	3	6	IronStrength	3	0 or cross-train	6
10	0 or cross-train	3	4	2	0	2	10-K

Intermediate: Moving Up

WEEK	MONDAY	TUESDAY	WEDNESDAY	THURSDAY	FRIDAY	SATURDAY	SUNDAY
1	0 or cross-train	4	6	IronStrength	3–4	0 or cross-train	6–7
2	0 or cross-train	4	6	IronStrength	3–4	0 or cross-train	6
3	0 or cross-train	4–5	6	IronStrength	4	0 or cross-train	6–7
4	0 or cross-train	4–5	7–8	IronStrength	4	0 or cross-train	6
5	0 or cross-train	5	7–8	IronStrength	4	0 or cross-train	7–9
6	0 or cross-train	5–6	7–8	IronStrength	4	0 or cross-train	6
7	0 or cross-train	5–6	8	IronStrength	4	0 or cross-train	9–10

WEEK	MONDAY	TUESDAY	WEDNESDAY	THURSDAY	FRIDAY	SATURDAY	SUNDAY
8	0 or cross-train	4	8	IronStrength	4	0 or cross-train	6
9	0 or cross-train	4	7–8	IronStrength	4	0 or cross-train	6
10	0 or cross-train	3	6	2	0	2	10-K

Advanced: At the Front of the Pack

WEEK	MONDAY	TUESDAY	WEDNESDAY	THURSDAY	FRIDAY	SATURDAY	SUNDAY
1	0–2 or cross-train	4–6	6	IronStrength	4	0–3 or cross-train	6–8
2	0–2 or cross-train	4–6	6	IronStrength	4	0–3 or cross-train	6
3	0–2 or cross-train	4–6	7–8	IronStrength	4–5	0–3 or cross-train	6–8
4	0–2 or cross-train	6	7–8	IronStrength	4–5	0–3 or cross-train	6
5	0–2 or cross-train	6	8	IronStrength	5	0–3 or cross-train	8–10
6	0–2 or cross-train	6	8	IronStrength	5	0–3 or cross-train	6
7	0–2 or cross-train	6	8	IronStrength	5	0–3 or cross-train	10–12
8	0–2 or cross-train	6	8	IronStrength	6	0–3 or cross-train	8
9	0–2 or cross-train	4–6	7–8	IronStrength	6	0–3 or cross-train	6
10	0 or cross-train	4	6	0–2	0	2–3	10-K

THE HALF-MARATHON

Beginner: Just Getting Started

WEEK	MONDAY	TUESDAY	WEDNESDAY	THURSDAY	FRIDAY	SATURDAY	SUNDAY
1	0 or cross-train	3	6	IronStrength	3–4	0 or cross-train	6–8
2	0 or cross-train	3	6	IronStrength	3–4	0 or cross-train	6
3	0 or cross-train	3	6–7	IronStrength	3–4	0 or cross-train	8–10
4	0 or cross-train	3–4	6–7	IronStrength	3–4	0 or cross-train	6–8
5	0 or cross-train	3–4	7	IronStrength	4	0 or cross-train	10
6	0 or cross-train	3–4	7	IronStrength	4	0 or cross-train	8
7	0 or cross-train	3–4	7–8	IronStrength	4	0 or cross-train	10–12
8	0 or cross-train	3–4	5–6	IronStrength	4	0 or cross-train	8
9	0 or cross-train	3–4	7–8	IronStrength	4	0 or cross-train	12–14
10	0 or cross-train	3–4	8	IronStrength	4	0 or cross-train	8
11	0 or cross-train	3–4	6–7	IronStrength	3–4	0 or cross-train	6–8
12	0 or cross-train	3	6	3	0	2	HALF

Intermediate: Moving Up

WEEK	MONDAY	TUESDAY	WEDNESDAY	THURSDAY	FRIDAY	SATURDAY	SUNDAY
1	0–3 or cross-train	4–6	6–7	IronStrength	4	0 or cross-train	8–10
2	0–3 or cross-train	4–6	6–7	IronStrength	4	0 or cross-train	7
3	0–3 or cross-train	4–6	7–8	IronStrength	4–6	0 or cross-train	10–12
4	0–3 or cross-train	4–6	7–8	IronStrength	4–6	0 or cross-train	8
5	0–3 or cross-train	4–6	8	IronStrength	5–6	0 or cross-train	12–14

WEEK	MONDAY	TUESDAY	WEDNESDAY	THURSDAY	FRIDAY	SATURDAY	SUNDAY
6	0–3 or cross-train	4–6	8	IronStrength	5–6	0 or cross-train	9
7	0–3 or cross-train	4–6	8	IronStrength	5–6	0 or cross-train	14–16
8	0–3 or cross-train	4–6	6	IronStrength	5–6	0 or cross-train	9–10
9	0–3 or cross-train	4–6	8	IronStrength	5–6	0 or cross-train	16–18
10	0–3 or cross-train	5	8–9	IronStrength	5	0 or cross-train	10–12
11	0–3 or cross-train	4	6–8	IronStrength	4	0 or cross-train	8
12	0–3 or cross-train	4	6	3	0	2	HALF

Advanced: At the Front of the Pack

WEEK	MONDAY	TUESDAY	WEDNESDAY	THURSDAY	FRIDAY	SATURDAY	SUNDAY
1	0–3 or cross-train	4–5	7	IronStrength	4–5	0–3 or cross-train	10
2	0–3 or cross-train	4–5	7–8	IronStrength	4–5	0–3 or cross-train	7
3	0–3 or cross-train	5–6	8	IronStrength	5–6	0–3 or cross-train	12
4	0–3 or cross-train	5–6	8	IronStrength	5–6	0–3 or cross-train	9
5	0–3 or cross-train	6–7	8–9	IronStrength	6–7	0–3 or cross-train	14
6	0–3 or cross-train	6–7	8–10	IronStrength	6–7	0–3 or cross-train	9
7	0–3 or cross-train	6–7	8–10	IronStrength	6–7	0–3 or cross-train	16
8	0–3 or cross-train	6–7	7	IronStrength	6–7	0–3 or cross-train	10
9	0–3 or cross-train	6–7	9–10	IronStrength	6–7	0–3 or cross-train	18
10	0–3 or cross-train	6	10	IronStrength	6	0–3 or cross-train	12
11	0–3 or cross-train	5	8	IronStrength	5	0–3 or cross-train	8
12	0–3 or cross-train	5	6–8	3	0	2	HALF

THE MARATHON

Beginner: Just Getting Started

WEEK	MONDAY	TUESDAY	WEDNESDAY	THURSDAY	FRIDAY	SATURDAY	SUNDAY
1	0 or cross-train	3	6	IronStrength	3–4	0 or cross-train	6–8
2	0 or cross-train	3	6	IronStrength	3–4	0 or cross-train	6
3	0 or cross-train	3	6–7	IronStrength	3–4	0 or cross-train	8–10
4	0 or cross-train	3–4	6–7	IronStrength	3–4	0 or cross-train	6–8
5	0 or cross-train	3–4	7	IronStrength	4	0 or cross-train	10
6	0 or cross-train	3–4	7	IronStrength	4	0 or cross-train	8
7	0 or cross-train	3–4	7–8	IronStrength	4	0 or cross-train	12
8	0 or cross-train	3–4	5–6	IronStrength	4	0 or cross-train	8
9	0 or cross-train	3–4	7–8	IronStrength	4	0 or cross-train	15
10	0 or cross-train	3–4	6–7	IronStrength	4	0 or cross-train	8
11	0 or cross-train	3	6	3	0	2	HALF
12	0 or cross-train	0–3	4	IronStrength	3	0 or cross-train	8–10
13	0–3 or cross-train	3	6	IronStrength	4	0 or cross-train	16–18
14	0–3 or cross-train	3–4	8	IronStrength	4	0 or cross-train	12
15	0–3 or cross-train	3–4	9	IronStrength	4	0 or cross-train	20
16	0–3 or cross-train	3–4	9–10	IronStrength	3	0 or cross-train	12
17	0–3 or cross-train	3	7	IronStrength	3	0 or cross-train	8*
18	0–3 or cross-train	3	6	0–3	0	2	MARATHON
19	0	0 or cross-train	3	0	3	0 or cross-train	3–5

*8-mile run or 3-mile warmup, 5-K race, and 2-mile cooldown

Intermediate: Moving Up

WEEK	MONDAY	TUESDAY	WEDNESDAY	THURSDAY	FRIDAY	SATURDAY	SUNDAY
1	0–3 or cross-train	4–6	6–7	IronStrength	4	0 or cross-train	8–10
2	0–3 or cross-train	4–6	6–7	IronStrength	4	0 or cross-train	7
3	0–3 or cross-train	4–6	7–8	IronStrength	4–6	0 or cross-train	10–12
4	0–3 or cross-train	4–6	7–8	IronStrength	4–6	0 or cross-train	8
5	0–3 or cross-train	4–6	8	IronStrength	5–6	0 or cross-train	12–14
6	0–3 or cross-train	4–6	8	IronStrength	5–6	0 or cross-train	9
7	0–3 or cross-train	4–6	8	IronStrength	5–6	0 or cross-train	14–16
8	0–3 or cross-train	4–6	6	IronStrength	5–6	0 or cross-train	9–10
9	0–3 or cross-train	4–6	8	IronStrength	5–6	0 or cross-train	16–18
10	0–3 or cross-train	4	6–8	IronStrength	5	0 or cross-train	8
11	0–3 or cross-train	4	6	3	0	2	HALF
12	0–3 or cross-train	0–3	4	IronStrength	3	0 or cross-train	8–10
13	0–3 or cross-train	4	6	IronStrength	5	0 or cross-train	18–20
14	0–3 or cross-train	4–6	9	IronStrength	5–6	0 or cross-train	12
15	0–3 or cross-train	4–6	9	IronStrength	5–6	0 or cross-train	20
16	0–3 or cross-train	4–6	9–10	0–3 plus IronStrength	5–6	0 or cross-train	15
17	0–3 or cross-train	4	7	IronStrength	4	0 or cross-train	8*
18	0–3 or cross-train	4	6	3	0	2	MARATHON
19	0	0 or cross-train	3	0	3	0 or cross-train	3–5

*8-mile run or 3-mile warmup, 5-K race, and 2-mile cooldown

Advanced: At the Front of the Pack

WEEK	MONDAY	TUESDAY	WEDNESDAY	THURSDAY	FRIDAY	SATURDAY	SUNDAY
1	0–3 or cross-train	4–5	7	IronStrength	4–5	0–3 or cross-train	10
2	0–3 or cross-train	4–5	7–8	IronStrength	4–5	0–3 or cross-train	7
3	0–3 or cross-train	5–6	8	IronStrength	5–6	0–3 or cross-train	12
4	0–3 or cross-train	5–6	8	IronStrength	5–6	0–3 or cross-train	9
5	0–3 or cross-train	6–7	8–9	IronStrength	6–7	0–3 or cross-train	14
6	0–3 or cross-train	6–7	8–10	IronStrength	6–7	0–3 or cross-train	9
7	0–3 or cross-train	6–7	8–10	IronStrength	6–7	0–3 or cross-train	16
8	0–3 or cross-train	6–7	7	IronStrength	6–7	0–3 or cross-train	10
9	0–3 or cross-train	6–7	9–10	IronStrength	6–7	0–3 or cross-train	18–20
10	0–3 or cross-train	5	0	IronStrength	6	0–3 or cross-train	8
11	0–3 or cross-train	5	6–8	3	0	2	HALF
12	0 or cross-train	0–3	4–6	IronStrength	3	0 or cross-train	8–10
13	0–3 or cross-train	3–5	6–8	IronStrength	6	0 or cross-train	18–20
14	0–3 or cross-train	6–7	10	IronStrength	6–7	0 or cross-train	12
15	0–3 or cross-train	6–7	11	IronStrength	6	0 or cross-train	20–22
16	0–3 or cross-train	6–7	11	IronStrength	6	0 or cross-train	15
17	0–3 or cross-train	6	8	IronStrength	6	0 or cross-train	8*
18	0–3 or cross-train	4	6	3	0	2	MARATHON
19	0	0 or cross-train	3	0	3	0 or cross-train	5

*8-mile run or 3-mile warmup, 5-K race, and 2-mile cooldown

ACKNOWLEDGMENTS

Dr. Jordan Metzl's Running Strong is a compilation of essential tips, secrets, and strategies that have kept me and my patients moving and injury-free for many years. This book and video series are the result of a team of many hardworking people, all of whom have helped make this project a reality.

First of all, I am deeply grateful to the entire team at *Runner's World* magazine. When video editor David Graf first wandered into my strength class 4 years ago, little did I know that after I kicked his butt, he would help me produce a series of videos that have become the IronStrength workout and the Inside the Doctor's Office series. From editor-in-chief David Willey to books editor Mark Weinstein to all the terrific employees at *Runner's World*, I am so honored to be counted among your ranks. Your dedication to the education of the running public is the best in the world, and I'm so appreciative of the chance to work with you.

The team at Rodale, top to bottom, is exceptional. For all my work in the past and all the work I will do in the future, I am thrilled to be associated with you.

I would also like to thank Claire Kowalchik, whose editorial skill, humor, and incredible talent helped me shape the day-to-day practice of treating runners into the publication before you. Claire, thank you for your tireless efforts to make *Dr. Jordan Metzl's Running Strong* accessible to everyone.

As the industry leader in orthopedics and sports medicine, my workplace, the Hospital for Special Surgery, has provided me with phenomenal educational and institutional support to treat, educate, research, and ultimately prevent injuries in thousands of runners. It is an honor to work among such outstanding colleagues and friends.

I am deeply appreciative to be part of the running community in New York City. From the New York Road Runners Club to the many running groups and clubs throughout the city, the community of New York runners is vibrant, each person always striving for his or her best. If you ever come run in New York, you will see what I mean.

Finally, my patients, family, and friends greatly enrich my ability to run my best life. From the hundreds of people who come to my IronStrength classes to my brothers who join me in triathlons and running races to my community of friends who make up my running posse, everyone who runs with me makes me better. Although running is an individual pursuit, the community of workout partners and friends in my life has blessed every aspect of my existence. I feel so truly lucky to have ended up among such loving, supportive people.

Running provides the joy of movement. If you run, you will be happier, healthier, and younger in body and mind. No matter how fast or how far, go for it!

My hope is that you will run strong wherever you are.

I look forward to seeing you on the road.

Jordan D. Metzl, MD
Hospital for Special Surgery
New York City

ABOUT THE AUTHORS

Jordan D. Metzl, MD, is a nationally known sports medicine physician at New York City's Hospital for Special Surgery. The author of *The Athlete's Book of Home Remedies* and *The Exercise Cure*, he is a frequent guest on *TODAY* and has completed 12 Ironman Triathlons and 32 marathons (and counting). Dr. Metzl completed sports medicine fellowships at Harvard Medical School and Vanderbilt University and regularly appears on New York magazine's "Best Doctors" list. He lives in New York City.

Claire Kowalchik has been running, writing, and editing for more than 20 years. She's completed countless road races and eight marathons, including twice running the Boston Marathon. Author of *The Complete Book of Running for Women* and the coauthor of *Running On Air* (with Budd Coates), she is also a former editor at *Runner's World* magazine, Prevention's Special Interest Publications, and *Diane*, a women's health and fitness publication from Curves International. She lives in Emmaus, Pennsylvania, with her sons, Michael and Benjamin Shimer.

INDEX

Boldface page references indicate illustrations. <u>Underscored</u> references indicate boxed text.

IronStrength workout (cont.)
    foam roller routine, 210–13,
        211–13
    in pregnancy, 281
    stretches, 208–9, **208–9**
    supersets, 201–6
ITB, **81**, 81–83, 115–16
ITB rolls, 87, **87**, 212, **212**
ITB/TFL stretches, 131, **131**

J

Joint cartilage, <u>18</u>
Jumping jacks, 199, **199**

K

Kegel exercises, 190
Kinetic chain
    described, 7–8
    imbalances, 22–23, 26–27
    role in running, 20–22
    steps to awesome, <u>22</u>
    strength, 8–9, 20, 197
Kneeling hip flexor stretches, 104,
    104
Knees, 75–93
    ailments, <u>76</u>, **76**, 76–86
        arthritis of the knee, <u>76</u>, **84**,
            84–86
        iliotibial band impingement
            syndrome, <u>76</u>, **81**, 81–83
        patellar tendonitis, <u>76</u>, **79**,
            79–80
        runner's knee, <u>76</u>, **76**, 77–78
    foam roller exercises, 87, **87**
    role in running, 21
    strength exercises, 88–93, **88–93**
Krebs cycle, 224, 226–27

L

Lactate, <u>226–27</u>, 226–28, <u>229</u>, 233
Lactate threshold, 227–28, 231
Lateral band walks, 92, **92**, 140,
    140

LDL cholesterol, 251–52, 254
Learning curve, 220, 226
Leg extension machine, 80
Leg extensions, 89, **89**
Legs
    lower, 57–74
        Achilles tendonitis, <u>58</u>, **59**,
            59–61
        ailments, <u>58</u>, 59–70
        anatomy, **58**
        calf strain, <u>58</u>, **68**, 68–70
        foam roller exercises, 72, **72**
        shin splints, <u>58</u>, **62**, 63–66, <u>67</u>
        strength exercises, 73–74,
            73–74
        stretches, 71, **71**
    upper, 95–110
        ailments, <u>97</u>, 98–103
        anatomy, 96, **96–97**
        middle-third hamstring strain,
            <u>97</u>, 100–101, **101**
        proximal hamstring strain, <u>97</u>,
            102, 102–3
        quadriceps strain, <u>97</u>, **98**,
            98–99
        strength exercises, 106–10,
            106–10
        stretches, 104–5, **104–5**
Legs down, 204, **204**
Liftoff, 28
Ligament, <u>18</u>, 36
Lip balm, 177
Lips, chapped, 177
Longevity, influence of exercise on,
    12
Long run, 232, 235–36
Lower back, 141–52
    ailments, <u>142</u>, 143–48
        arthritis of the spine, <u>142</u>,
            147–48
        discogenic back pain, <u>142</u>,
            145, 145–46
        muscle spasm, <u>142</u>, **143**,
            143–44
    anatomy, **142**
    foam roller exercises, 149, **149**
    strength exercises, 150–52,
        150–52
    stretches, 149, **149**

Lower-back rolls, 213, **213**
Lower-back spasm, <u>142</u>, **143**,
    143–44
Lower legs, 57–74
    ailments, <u>58</u>, 59–70
        Achilles tendonitis, <u>58</u>, **59**,
            59–61
        calf strain, <u>58</u>, **68**, 68–70
        shin splints, <u>58</u>, **62**, 63–66, <u>67</u>
    anatomy, **58**
    foam roller exercises, 72, **72**
    strength exercises, 73–74, **73–74**
    stretches, 71, **71**
Low side-to-side lunges, 91, **91**,
    137, **137**
Lunges, 55, **55**, 107, **107**
Lying glutes stretches, 105, **105**,
    132, **132**, 149, **149**
Lyme disease, <u>184</u>

M

Male runners, 282–83
Mantra, 242
Massage, 11–12, 15, 210, <u>215</u>,
    215–16
Max VO$_2$, <u>222</u>
Meals, number of, 256
Mechanics of running, 17–29
Mediterranean diet, 254–55
Melanoma, 188, 272
Menstrual cycle, 278, <u>278</u>
Mental strategies, 242–46
    breathing, <u>242</u>, 242–44
    centering, 243
    mind-body connection, 243–44,
        246
    relaxation techniques, 242, <u>242</u>,
        246
    visualization, <u>241</u>, 244–45
Metatarsals, 41, **41**, 44, 44–45,
    174
Middle-third hamstring strain, <u>97</u>,
    100–101, **101**
Midfoot strike, <u>24</u>, 27, 229, 231,
    264
Migraine, <u>155</u>, 162–63
Mileage, increasing, 237–38